SARS: A Case Study in Emerging Infections

SARS: A Case Study in Emerging Infections

EDITED BY

Angela R. McLean
University of Oxford, UK

Robert M. May
University of Oxford, UK

John Pattison
Department of Health, UK

Robin A. Weiss
University College London, UK

Originating from a Royal Society Discussion Meeting first published in Philosophical Transactions of the Royal Society B: Biological Sciences

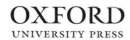

OXFORD
UNIVERSITY PRESS

OXFORD
UNIVERSITY PRESS

Great Clarendon Street, Oxford OX2 6DP

Oxford University Press is a department of the University of Oxford.
It furthers the University's objective of excellence in research, scholarship,
and education by publishing worldwide in

Oxford New York

Auckland Cape Town Dare es Salaam Hong Kong Karachi
Kuala Lumpur Madrid Melbourne Mexico City Nairobi
Shanghai Taipei Toronto New Delhi

With offices in

Argentina Austria Brazil Chile Czech Republic France Greece
Guatemala Hungary Italy Japan South Korea Poland Portugal
Singapore Switzerland Thailand Turkey Ukraine Vietnam

Published in the United States
by Oxford University Press Inc., New York

British Library Cataloging in Publication Data
(Data available)

Library of Congress Cataloging-in-Publication Data
SARS : a case study in emerging infections / edited by Angela McLean ... [et al.].
    p. cm.

  ISBN 0-19-856819-3 (alk. paper) – ISBN 0-19-856818-5 (alk. paper)   1. SARS
(Disease)–Epidemiology.   I. McLean, Angela.   II. Royal Society (Great Britain)
  RA644.S17S27 2005
  614.5′92–dc22   2004027494
ISBN 0-19-856818-5 (Hbk.)
ISBN 0-19-856819-3 (Pbk.)

10 9 8 7 6 5 4 3 2 1

Typeset by Newgen Imaging Systems (P) Ltd., Chennai, India
Printed in Great Britain on acid-free paper by Antony Rowe, Chippenham

Contents

Contributors

Roy M. Anderson, Department of Infectious Disease Epidemiology, Faculty of Medicine, Imperial College London, St Mary's Campus, Norfolk Place, London W2 1PG, UK.

Hazel Appleton, Centre for Infection, Health Protection Agency, 61 Colindale Avenue, London, NW9 5HT.

Ken Balderson, Department of Psychiatry, University of Toronto, Toronto, Canada.; St. Michael's Hospital, Toronto, Ontario, Canada.

Diana J. Bell, Centre for Ecology, Evolution and Conservation, School of Biological Sciences, University of East Anglia, Norwich NR4 7TJ.

Alison Bermingham, Centre for Infection, Health Protection Agency, 61 Colindale Avenue, London, NW9 5HT

D. Brockmann, Max-Planck-Institut für Strömungsforschung Bunsenstr. 10, 37073 Göttingen, Germany.

Robin M. Bush, Department of Ecology and Evolutionary Biology, 321 Steinhaus, University of California, Irvine, CA 92697, USA.

Christl A. Donnelly, Department of Infectious Disease Epidemiology, Faculty of Medicine, Imperial College London, St Mary's Campus, Norfolk Place, London W2 1PG, UK.

Neil M. Ferguson, Department of Infectious Disease Epidemiology, Faculty of Medicine, Imperial College London, St Mary's Campus, Norfolk Place, London W2 1PG, UK.

Calvin S. L. Fones, Psychological Medicine, National University of Singapore, Singapore.

Ron A. M. Fouchier, Institute of Virology, Erasmus University Rotterdam, Dr Molewaterplein 50, 3015 GE Rotterdam, The Netherlands.

Christophe Fraser, Department of Infectious Disease Epidemiology, Faculty of Medicine, Imperial College London, St Mary's Campus, Norfolk Place, London W2 1PG, UK.

Theo Geisel, Max-Planck-Institut für Strömungsforschung Bunsenstr. 10, 37073 Göttingen, Germany.

Azra C. Ghani, Department of Infectious Disease Epidemiology, Faculty of Medicine, Imperial College London, St Mary's Campus, Norfolk Place, London W2 1PG, UK.

David S. Goldbloom, Centre for Addiction and Mental Health, Toronto, Ontario, Canada; Department of Psychiatry, University of Toronto, Toronto, Canada.

Jim J. Gray, Enteric Virus Unit, Centre for Infection, Health Protection Agency, 61 Colindale Avenue, London, NW9 5HT.

Y. Guan, Department of Microbiology, The University of Hong Kong, Pokfulam, Hong Kong SAR, China.

Anthony J. Hedley, Sassoon Road, Faculty of Medicine Building, University of Hong Kong, Pokfulam, Hong Kong, China.

Paul P. Heinen, Centre for Infection, Health Protection Agency, 61 Colindale Avenue, London, NW9 5HT.

David L. Heymann, Former Executive Director of Communicable Diseases, current Special Representative of the Director General for Polio Eradication, POL, World Health Organisation, 20 Avenue Appia, 1211 Geneva 27, Switzerland.

Edward C. Holmes, Department of Zoology, University of Oxford, South Parks Road, Oxford OX1 3PS, UK.

Lars Hufnagel Max-Planck-Institut für Strömungsforschung Bunsenstr. 10, 37073 Göttingen, Germany.

Paul R. Hunter, School of Medicine, Health Policy and Practice, University of East Anglia, Norwich NR4 7TJ, UK.

Jonathan Hunter, Mount Sinai Hospital, Toronto, Ontario, Canada; Department of Psychiatry, University of Toronto, Toronto, Canada.

Miren Iturriza-Gómara, Enteric Virus Unit Centre for Infection, Health Protection Agency, 61 Colindale Avenue, London, NW9 5HT.

David Koh, Community Occupational and Family Medicine, National University of Singapore.

Thijs Kuiken, Institute of Virology, Erasmus University Rotterdam, Dr Molewaterplein 50, 3015 GE Rotterdam, The Netherlands.

Tai H. Lam, Sassoon Road, Faculty of Medicine Building, University of Hong Kong, Pokfulam, Hong Kong, China.

William J. Lancee, Mount Sinai Hospital, Toronto, Ontario, Canada.; Department of Psychiatry, University of Toronto, Toronto, Canada.

Molyn Leszcz, Mount Sinai Hospital, Toronto, Ontario, Canada.; Department of Psychiatry, University of Toronto, Toronto, Canada.

Gabriel M. Leung, Sassoon Road, Faculty of Medicine Building, University of Hong Kong, Pokfulam, Hong Kong, China.

Robert Maunder, Mount Sinai Hospital, Toronto, Ontario, Canada., Department of Psychiatry, University of Toronto, Toronto, Canada.

Robert M. May, Department of Zoology, University of Oxford, South Parks Road, Oxford OX1 3PS, UK

Angela R. McLean, Zoology Department, Oxford University, South Parks Road, Oxford OX1 3PS UK.

Anthony J. McMichael, National Centre for Epidemiology and Population Health, The Australian National University, Canberra, Australia.

Onora O'Neill, Newnham College, Cambridge, CB3 9DF.

Ab D. M. E. Osterhaus, Institute of Virology, Erasmus University Rotterdam, Dr Molewaterplein 50, 3015 GE Rotterdam, The Netherlands.

John Pattison, Department of Health, Richmond House, Whitehall, London SW1A 2NS, UK.

J. S. Malik Peiris, Department of Microbiology, The University of Hong Kong, Pokfulam, Hong Kong SAR China.

Patricia M. Petryshen, St. Michael's Hospital, Toronto, Ontario, Canada.

Andrew Rambaut, Department of Zoology, University of Oxford, South Parks Road, Oxford OX1 3PS, UK.

Steven Riley, Department of Infectious Disease Epidemiology, Faculty of Medicine, Imperial College London, St Mary's Campus, Norfolk Place, London W2 1PG, UK.

Scott Roberton, Centre for Ecology, Evolution and Conservation, School of Biological Sciences, University of East Anglia, Norwich NR4 7TJ.

Sean B. Rourke, Department of Psychiatry, University of Toronto, Toronto, Canada.; St. Michael's Hospital, Toronto, Ontario, Canada.

Rosalie Steinberg, Mount Sinai Hospital, Toronto, Ontario, Canada; Department of Psychiatry, University of Toronto, Toronto, Canada.

Donald Wasylenki, Department of Psychiatry, University of Toronto, Toronto, Canada; St Michael's Hospital, Toronto, Ontario, Canada.

Robin A. Weiss, Division of Infection and Immunity, University College London, 46 Cleveland Street, London, W1T 4JF, UK.

Maria C. Zambon, Enteric, Respiratory and Neurological Laboratory, Centre for Infection, Health Protection Agency, 61, Colindale Avenue, London NW9 5HT.

Guangqiao Zeng, Guangzhou Institute of Respiratory Diseases, Guangzhou China 510120.

Nanshan Zhong, Guangzhou Institute of Respiratory Diseases, Guangzhou China 510120.

List of Abbreviations

CDC	Centre for Disease control
CFR	case fatality rate
CJD	Creutzfeldt–Jakob Disease
CPAP	continuous positive airway
CPE	cytopathic effect
GEIS	Global Emerging Infections Surveillance and Response System
GHQ	general health questionnaire
GOARN	Global Outbreak Alert and Response Network
GPHIN	Global Public Health Intelligence Network
hMPV	human metapneumovirus
IHR	International Health Regulations
Lao PDR	Lao People's Democratic Republic
RDS	Respiratory distress syndrome
RT-PCR	reverse transcription–polymerase chain reaction
SARS	severe acute respiratory syndrome
SARS-CoV	severe acute respiratory syndrome coronavirus
SIR	susceptible-infected recovered frameworks
SSC	Species Survival Commission
SSE	super-spreading event
WHO	World Health Organization

CHAPTER 1

Introduction

Angela R. McLean, Robert M. May, John Pattison, and Robin A. Weiss

The rapid global spread of Severe Acute Respiratory Syndrome (SARS) during the winter of 2003 served as a wake-up call to the world that emerging infections are a problem we all share. Living in rich countries with good healthcare systems does not necessarily protect us from the dangers posed by newly emerging, life-threatening infections. The SARS epidemic tested global preparedness for dealing with such a new infectious agent and very naturally raised the questions: how did we do and what did we learn?

Emerging infections are defined as infections that are increasing in incidence (e.g. tuberculosis), newly identified agents thought to have been circulating for some time (e.g. *Helicobacter pylori*) or genuinely novel infectious agents that have only recently spread into the human population (e.g. HIV and SARS). This book is concerned with this third group of novel emerging infections. Emerging infections are more than just a current biological fashion. The bitter ongoing experience of AIDS and the looming threat of an influenza pandemic teach us that the control of infectious disease is a problem we have not yet solved. It is a problem that needs to be addressed by a broad community. Scientists, policy-makers, and healthcare workers all need to be prepared, but prepared to do what? The purpose of this book is to use SARS as a case study of the tasks that must be addressed by a community that wishes to prepare for further emerging infections.

The book has four parts. Central sections on the biology and transmission of SARS are sandwiched between an opening section on horizon scanning and a closing section on infection control.

Horizon scanning is an often-used, but ill-defined term. In essence it addresses the question

'What is coming next?' This is a question that we cannot answer with any confidence. We can, however, make sensible statements about the environmental and social changes that have facilitated the emergence of novel agents in the past. We can also inspect the range of recently emerged infections and ask what genetic properties their causal agents share. Finally, we can look back at the ecology and evolution of influenza and seek insight from data on the best documented of zoonotic infections. These three tasks are described in chapters on environmental change by Tony McMichael (Chapter 2), viral evolutionary genetics by Eddie Holmes and Andrew Rambaut (Chapter 3), and influenza by Robin Bush (Chapter 4).

When a novel infection emerges, it takes time before individual case reports coalesce into a picture of an outbreak of something new. There then follow urgent tasks of case definition, identification of the causative agent, and the rapid development of diagnostic tools. The stories of how these tasks were addressed are described in four chapters. Nanshan Zhong and Guangqiao Zeng describe the early outbreak of SARS in late 2002 that took place in Guangdong Province in Mainland China (Chapter 5). Malik Peiris and Yi Guan describe the unfolding of events in Hong Kong (Chapter 6), Ab Osterhaus and co-authors describe how Koch's postulates were established (Chapter 7) and Maria Zambon and co-authors describe the development of molecular and serological diagnostic tools (Chapter 8).

Once it is clear that a new infectious agent is spreading, the task of controlling that spread becomes paramount. The question of the original source of the infectious agent arises very naturally.

It has become clear that coronaviruses closely related to SARS-CoV can be isolated from wild animals being sold for meat in markets in China. Diana Bell and co-authors (Chapter 9) present an overview of the impact of this international trade in wildlife for food and raises important questions about how it can best be monitored and controlled. As information about the modes and rates of spread is gathered it becomes possible to make rational statements about the interventions that are most likely to bring transmission under control. Anderson and co-authors (Chapter 10) enumerate the types of information that need to be collated and show how they can be used to design effective local control measures. The spread of SARS dramatically illustrated the role of global air travel in moving a new agent all across the world. Dirk Brockmann and co-authors (Chapter 11) present new mathematical models of such spread and use them to compare the impact of different interventions.

The fourth section of this book addresses issues of planning and preparedness. For the healthcare workers whose job it was to keep hospitals running under strict regimes for infection control, it was a time of enormous stress. Robert Maunder and co-authors (Chapter 13) describe studies that show that over one-third of healthcare workers in Toronto suffered a high degree of stress during the SARS outbreak there. David Heymann (Chapter 12) describes the World Health Organization's (WHO) role in coordinating the global response to SARS. Finally there is a discussion from Onora O'Neill (Chapter 14) about the rights and wrongs of individual freedoms in a society threatened with an infectious disease that can only be controlled by quarantine.

The book ends with an overview by two of us, Robin Weiss and Angela McLean (Chapter 15) which asks 'What have we learnt from SARS?' On an optimistic note, there have clearly been great triumphs in the use of modern laboratory and communications techniques to identify the causative agents with breathtaking speed. But on a more sombre note, we cannot expect every emerging infection to be successfully controlled with quarantine measures and infection control in hospitals. Above all, we are painfully aware that we can expect further unpleasant surprises.

From these varied contributions four themes arise on which there is broad consensus. First, SARS could have been very much worse. Many authors expressed fear of the emergence of a novel strain of influenza capable of pandemic spread. Second, mass air travel has created a global village, in which apparently distant health problems in obscure parts of China are actually health problems that can rapidly be shared by all of us. Third, the emergence of novel infectious agents can be broken down into several steps, with genetic changes in the agent and ecological changes in the human hosts playing different roles at each step. Finally, the study of novel emerging infections is beset with uncertainties. These uncertainties are of two broad types: 'peacetime' uncertainties about how to predict what will happen next, and 'outbreak' uncertainties about what is happening right at the moment.

Several authors refer to the pandemic influenza as the greatest threat among emerging infections. Malik Peiris (Chapter 6) points out that the high, and early, infectiousness of influenza would make it much harder to control than SARS proved to be. Anderson (Chapter 10) elaborates this point with a mathematical model. In his description of the WHO's response to SARS (Chapter 12) David Heymann relates that in early February 2003 their greatest fear was that they were witnessing the emergence of a new strain of influenza virus. As Robin Weiss and Angela McLean point out in the concluding comments (Chapter 15) humankind had a lucky escape in the SARS epidemic because patients were not very infectious before they were symptomatic.

Globalization through air travel is a second topic referred to by many authors. Dirk Brockmann's work (Chapter 11) specifically focuses on the issue and uses data on passenger movements to explore the impact of different types of travel ban. The models presented there illustrate rather starkly the point often made that because of globalization, an inadequate response to a public health emergency in one country can cause public health emergencies across the world.

The multi-step nature of the emergence of a novel infection is first referred to by Tony McMichael (Chapter 2). He describes how a novel infectious agent must first cross the species barrier into humans and then be able to spread among the human population. Environmental changes that allow new contacts with previously isolated infectious agents encourage the first step. Demographic changes that increase the propensity for humans to pass infections between each other encourage the second. In Chapter 3 Eddie Holmes points out that genetic changes in the infecting agent must also pass through the same two steps, the ability to infect a human at all, followed by the ability to transmit from one human to another. Almost every other chapter touches on these issues. Several cite examples of viruses that make the first step and infect humans (avian influenzas and probably coronaviruses that are cross reactive with SARS) but do not go on to transmit from human-to-human. Other chapters refer to socio-economic changes in Southeast Asian countries that predispose their populations to novel zoonotic infections. Increased commercialization of the bush-meat trade makes new opportunities for the first step while increased density and mobility of the human population makes onward spread easier.

The fourth consensus among these chapters is that SARS and other novel emerging infections present us with great uncertainties. The 'peace-time' uncertainties concern attempts to predict what will emerge next. We know so little about what allows a virus to cross a species barrier that we are currently incapable of predicting which animal viruses pose the greatest threat. More fundamentally, we know very little at all about the infectious agents that wild animals carry. As for the process by which novel human pathogens arise, Robin Bush lucidly warns that even the widely cited hypothesis about the mixing of human and avian influenza virus strains in pigs is not well supported by the available data. In short, we do not know what is out there, and we do not know which of the things that are out there is most likely to pose a new problem.

The uncertainties that arise during an outbreak paint a more encouraging picture, as they can be resolved as the outbreak progresses. The first step in an outbreak is to identify the fact that a new clinical entity has arisen. In Chapter 6, Malik Peiris describes how hard this was in Hong Kong where 55–75 cases of community-acquired pneumonia that need intensive care occur every month. Identification of a new clinical entity triggers a search for the causative agent. Again this is fraught with difficulties, especially when the case definition is broad enough that not all suspect cases will harbour the novel agent. Ab Osterhaus (Chapter 7) describes how human meta-pneumovirus was isolated from many suspected SARS cases and was therefore a strong suspect as the causative agent for some time. The best way to treat SARS patients is an uncertainty that was not resolved over the course of the epidemic. For the general public the most worrying questions about a new infection are its routes and rates of spread. The impact of these uncertainties is particularly acute. Both the general public and healthcare workers seek reliable information about the degree of risk they face at a time when no such information exists. In Chapter 13, Robert Maunder describes how such uncertainties provide 'a volatile fuel for anxiety'. Until the routes and rates of spread are understood it is very difficult for policy-makers to design intervention programmes. In Chapter 14 Onora O'Neill points out that the associated problem of assessing the magnitude of any risk makes it very difficult to establish the legitimate scope of compulsory measures to control infection.

Uncertainty as a consensus state may seem a dismal kind of science. But it is helpful to be quite clear of what we are most uncertain about. We can also be encouraged that many of the immediate uncertainties that arose during the SARS outbreak were resolved quite quickly. The broader tasks of understanding the processes that underlie the emergence of novel infections offer a worthy challenge that will not be solved so quickly.

CHAPTER 2

Environmental and social influences on emerging infectious diseases: past, present, and future

Anthony J. McMichael

2.1 Summary

The processes of worldwide human population dispersal over the past 50,000–100,000 years, along with cultural evolution and inter-population contacts, have had profound consequences for the relationship between *Homo sapiens* and the microbiological world. In particular, there have been several major transitions at key junctures in human history, each entailing the emergence of various new or unfamiliar infectious diseases.

There have been three main historical transitions since the advent of agriculture and livestock herding, which began around 10,000 years ago. These transitions occurred when: (1) early agrarian-based settlements enabled enzootic microbes to cross the species barrier and make contact with *Homo sapiens*; (2) early Eurasian civilizations came into military and commercial contact around 3000–2000 years ago, thereby swapping their dominant infectious agents; and (3) European expansionism, over the past five centuries, caused the transoceanic spread of often lethal infectious diseases.

Today, we are living through the fourth of these great transitions, extending this time to global scale. The contemporary spread and increased liability of various infectious diseases, new and old, reflect the combined and increasingly widespread impacts of demographic, commercial, environmental, behavioural, technological, and other rapid changes in human ecology. Modern clinical medicine, via blood transfusion, organ transplantation, and hypodermic syringes, has created new opportunities for microbes, contributing to rises in hepatitis C, HIV/AIDS, and several other viral infections. Meanwhile, injudicious use of antibiotics has resulted, unusually, in human actions actually increasing genetic 'biodiversity'.

As with the previous human–microbe transitions, a new equilibrium state may lie ahead. However, that state will certainly not entail a world free of infectious diseases. A mature and sustainable form of human ecology must accommodate the need for, and the needs of, the microbial species that help to make up the interdependent system of Life on Earth. Humans and microbes are not 'at war' (as much popular literature suggests). Rather, both parties are engaged in amoral, self-interested, coevolutionary struggle. We need to understand better, and therefore anticipate, the dynamics of that process.

2.2 Introduction

Over the past decade, there has been renewed public and official concern about infectious disease as a resurgent public health threat. That concern has been coupled, though, with some surprise. After all, we modern citizens are protected by a plethora of vaccinations and antibiotics. We live in hygienic homes with sweet-smelling toilet bowls, and we eat pressure-packed sterilized foods. Surely germ-free Nirvana is near. Yet, in the past quarter century we have encountered the emergence of many new or newly identified infectious diseases, including Legionnaire's disease, Lyme disease, HIV/AIDS, hepatitis C, Ebola virus, human 'mad cow disease' (variant CJD), the Nipah virus, West Nile fever, and severe acute respiratory syndrome (SARS)—as well as resurgent infectious diseases such as tuberculosis, cholera, dengue fever, and malaria.

Public anxiety over the 'emergence and resurgence' of infectious diseases has been particularly prominent within the media-driven culture of the United States. Titles of some recent popular-science offerings by American authors include *The coming plague, The hot zone, Virus hunter*, and *Secret agents: the menace of emerging infections*. Military metaphors abound: we are under siege from microbes; germs are invaders; we brace for the next wave; we counter-attack with antibiotics. This them-versus-us perspective is misleading, of course; it inappropriately implies malign microbial intent. This fundamentally misrepresents the aeons-old ecological struggle in which microbes must engage for their survival. Microbes wish the infected host neither well nor ill. Their interest is in surviving and reproducing; biological detriment to the host is either incidental or, at worst, a means to the microbe's ends.

The prevailing ecological conditions in today's world are propitious for infectious disease agents. Human mobility and long-distance trade have increased; ever-larger cities, often girded with slums, have become highways for microbial traffic; poverty perpetuates vulnerability to infectious disease; and sexual practices, drug injecting, intensified food production, and much modern medical technology all create new opportunities for microbial opportunism. Chapter 11 of this book presents new mathematical models of the impact of global air travel on the spread of emerging infections. A newer, larger-scale, influence on patterns of infectious disease is that of global climate change, widespread land-use changes, biodiversity losses, and other global environmental changes that characterize the contemporary world (Patz and Confalonieri 2004). Meanwhile, widespread antibiotic resistance, especially of staphylococci, streptococci, and enterococci, has followed our injudicious over-use of these drugs.

Cholera provides an instructive example of how modern conditions, operating at large scale, can affect infectious diseases. The ancestral home of cholera was the Ganges delta, in India, where epidemics of a cholera-like disease have been described over the past four centuries. Since the early 1960s, a major, continuing, pandemic of cholera has occurred. This is the seventh pandemic since cholera (reinforced with a newly acquired toxin-producing gene) first extended its range beyond South Asia in 1817. That initial spread occurred in the wake of the Great Kumbh religious festival in the Upper Ganges, in which pilgrims from all over India came annually to bathe in the sacred waters. Their subsequent dispersal, and contacts with British troops mobilizing in the Northwest Frontier region, led to a cholera pandemic that spread from India to the Arabian Peninsula and along the trade routes to Africa and the Mediterranean coast.

In the early 1830s, the faster-travelling steamboats enabled cholera to cross the Atlantic. The disease reached North America in 1832, arriving first in Montreal, New York, and Philadelphia. In the United States, the disease spread rapidly around the coastline and inland via major rivers. Public hysteria, fanned by local newspaper stories, spread rapidly.

This seventh pandemic has reached further than ever before, affecting Asia, Europe, Africa, North America, and Latin America. It began in 1961 and is by far the longest lasting pandemic to date (Lee and Dodgson 2000; WHO 2003*a*). This pandemic entails the El Tor strain, which, in mid-twentieth century, replaced the more lethal classical biotype of the nineteenth-century pandemics. However, the extraordinary scale of this pandemic seems to reflect much more than the biology of the bacterium. Rather, it appears to reflect the greatly increased volume of human movement between continents, the greater rapidity and distance of modern shipping-based trade, increased nutrient enrichment of coastal and estuarine waters by phosphates and nitrates in run-off water (which enhances the growth of vibrio-harbouring phytoplankton and zooplankton), and proliferation of urban slums without access to safe drinking water. That is, today's world has become a more conducive culture medium for the cholera bacterium.

Cholera, however, is a well-established and familiar disease. Our main interest, here, is in the appearance and spread of new, 'emerging', infectious diseases. However, note that the usage of this word 'emerging' has been somewhat ambiguous. In 1992, the US Institute of Medicine defined 'emerging' as subsuming three things:

(1) Established infectious diseases undergoing increased incidence;
(2) Newly discovered infections;
(3) Newly evolving (newly occurring) infections.

In the wake of the dramatic outbreak and spread of SARS in 2003, can we better understand the social, environmental, and related factors that potentiate the appearance of *new* infectious disease? Such understanding should help us anticipate any such future risks as human ecology—social, environmental, technological, and behavioural—continues to change.

2.3 Learning from emerging infections

Many new infectious diseases do not develop into serious public health problems (McMichael 2001). Some do little more than establish a toehold at the margins of human society. Others flicker sporadically. Some, such as the 'English Sweats' of the sixteenth century, may circulate for decades and then apparently disappear. We cannot know, in advance, what the future trajectory of a new infectious disease will be. Twenty years after the initial spread of HIV/AIDS we are aghast at the burgeoning scale of the pandemic. Meanwhile, the study of these emerging diseases can increase our understanding of the dynamics and ecology of infectious diseases and of diverse adaptation mechanisms that boost the survival or spread of pathogens.

The science of emerging infections used to be a lot simpler. In the words of the biblical Old Testament:

The Lord shall smite thee with a consumption, and with a fever, and with an inflammation, and with an extreme burning. (Deuteronomy 28: 22)

Indeed, when wrathful, the Lord was reportedly partial to quite a bit of smiting. Strange and often fatal diseases were thus dispensed as Divine Retribution.

The Revelation of St John the Divine—part of the Apocrypha that follows the Christian Bible's New Testament, and written ca. AD 100—gives a vivid account of these oft-dramatic afflictions of human societies. St John describes the Four Horsemen of the Apocalypse, the fourth (Pestilence, riding on a white horse) being the harbinger of near-certain death.

The four horsemen—war, Conquest, Famine, and Pestilence—are instructive in another sense. Two millennia ago in the eastern Mediterranean region, these were the four main recurring scourges of human happiness, health, and survival. As public health threats, they are all conceptualized in population-level terms. An individual may be starving or malnourished, but it is the population that experiences famine. An individual may contract an infection, but it is pestilence that afflicts the population. That is, these terms are attuned to the idea of population-based phenomena as determinants of health and survival. Regrettably, this perspective is often missing in contemporary discussion of the determinants of health (McMichael 2002).

The contemporary discussion should therefore give greater emphasis to understanding infectious disease within an ecological framework. It cannot be mere chance that there has been an upturn in the tempo of new and spreading infectious disease in recent decades. What, then, are the relative roles of changes in environmental and social conditions in the emergence of infectious diseases?

The word 'environmental' refers, here, to the physical circumstances of contact between pathogen and human. Environments can change at the micro-, meso-, and macro-scales. 'Social' encompasses group and individual-level behaviours, contact networks, cultural practices, choices of technology, and the distribution of advantage/disadvantage and related variations in vulnerability.

2.4 The process of 'emergence'

The primary 'environmental' event that initiates a new human infection is a novel physical contact between potential pathogen and human. The infectious agent mostly derives from an animal source, though some derive from the soil. A particular requirement, usually, is that the potential pathogen is a mutated strain that, fortuitously (for the microbe), has become better able to colonize and survive in the human host.

The subsequent persistence and spread of the 'new' infectious disease may depend on both environmental and social factors. These include:

(1) demographic characteristics and processes, human mobility, etc.;
(2) land use, other environmental changes, encroachment on new environments;
(3) consumption behaviours (eating, drinking, and, more generally, culinary culture);
(4) other behaviours (sexual contacts, IV drug use, hospital procedures, etc.);
(5) host condition (malnutrition, diabetes, immune status, etc.).

An example of an emerging disease that primarily reflects recent social–technological change is hepatitis C. This previously unknown hepatitis virus was identified in 1989, and may have been quietly circulating in humans for a very long time. The advent of illicit intravenous drug use, and of blood transfusion, has led to the wider spread and recognition of this virus.

The resurgence of several previously well-established infectious diseases—such as cholera, malaria, tuberculosis, and diphtheria (in 1990s Russia)—has been primarily attributable to changes in social conditions and behaviours. These include poverty, crowding, and the weakening of public health infrastructure. Indeed, this is an old, continuing story. Historically, epidemics have often accompanied periods of great social and demographic change. Examples include the bubonic plague in fourteenth-century Europe following the privations and poverty of the feudal system, exacerbated by several decades of miserable weather and crop failures; the scourges of tuberculosis, smallpox, and cholera in the squalid, crowded cities of nineteenth-century England; and the ravages of the Spanish influenza following the chaos of the First World War.

Today, various larger-scale environmental changes, both physical and ecological, are also influencing the resurgence of some infectious diseases. For example, the World Health Organization has recently estimated that about 6–7% of malaria in some parts of the world is attributable to the climate change that has occurred during the past quarter of a century (McMichael *et al.* in press).

2.5 Historical transitions, past and present

During many millennia of human dispersal around the world, cultural evolution, and increasing contact between populations, several distinct transitions in human ecology and in inter-population interactions have profoundly influenced the patterns of infectious disease. The main transitions have been, first, a prolonged prehistoric transition associated with hominid evolution and changing dietary and survival behaviours, and second a sequence of historic transitions:

(1) Local: ca. 5000–10,000 years ago;
(2) Continental: ca. 1000–3000 years ago;
(3) Intercontinental: from ca. AD 1500;
(4) Global: current.

The prehistoric transition began, several million years ago, with the move by australopithecines from tree dwelling to savannah. This entailed changes in exposures to mosquito and tick species. Likewise, the growing reliance of early *Homo* species on meat eating, from ca. 2 million years ago, and associated activities such as the use of animal skins and fur, would have increased exposure to enzootic pathogens and their vectors (including lice). The subsequent radiation of these upright-walking hunter-gatherers into unfamiliar environments would have exposed them to various new parasites.

This early transition illustrates the inter-relationship between the behavioural, social, and environmental domains, as joint influences on the emergence of infectious diseases. Selection pressures caused evolution of human behaviours, especially the move to a ground-dwelling upright-walking existence. This, in turn, entailed various environmental changes—such as exposure to different, low-flying, species of mosquitoes. There were also consequent changes in social relationships, in family and tribal groupings, and in patterns of day-to-day interaction between these hunter-gatherer hominids. Clearly, attempts to differentiate environmental and social influences on emerging infectious diseases will often be somewhat misplaced.

The opportunities for infectious disease agents were, however, severely limited in hunter-gatherer humans. Local communities were small, and these wandering bands made only occasional contact with one another. Human-adapted pathogens that caused acute disease could not have survived within such small groupings. The dominant infections would have been unhurried chronic infections (including parasitic worms and helminths), occasional zoonotic infections (such as rabies), and some viral infectious agents (such as the herpes virus family, the papovaviruses and the papilloma viruses) that had co-evolved with primates, hominids, and early humans (Weiss 2001).

Subsequently, following the initial emergence of agriculture and livestock herding, which began ca. 10,000 years ago in the eastern Mediterranean region, there have been three great historical transitions in human–microbe relationships. They occurred on an increasingly large scale and have been well described by the historian William McNeill (1975). These are 'historical' transitions in that they occurred after the advent of early writing, around 5000 years ago in Mesopotamia, which rendered recorded 'history' possible.

2.5.1 First historical transition

Conditions in early human settlements, which emerged during the period 5000–10,000 years ago, enabled various enzootic pathogens (often as serendipitous mutants) to enter the human species from husbanded animals and pest species (rodents, flies, etc.). Most such inter-species microbial contacts, with or without random mutations, would have failed. However, some of these inter-species crossovers, as more recently with the HIV, Nipah, and SARS viruses, would have succeeded. They were the progenitors of today's textbook infections: influenza, tuberculosis, leprosy, cholera, typhoid, smallpox, chicken pox, measles, typhus, malaria, plague, and many others. Table 2.1 (from

Table 2.1 Examples of human infectious diseases of animal origin, and apparent date(s) of species crossover

Disease	Microbe	Animal source	Date of crossover
Malaria	Parasite	Chimpanzee	ca. 8000 BCE
Measles	Virus	Sheep or goat	ca. 8000 BCE
Smallpox	Virus	Ruminant?	>2000 BCE
Tuberculosis	Mycobacterium	Ruminant?	>1000 BCE
Typhus	Rickettsia	Rodent	430 BCE and 1492 CE[a]
Plague	Bacterium	Rodent	541 CE, 1347 CE and 1665 CE
Dengue	Virus	Monkey	ca. 1000 CE
Yellow fever	Virus	Monkey	1641 CE
Spanish flu	Virus	Bird, pig	1918 CE
AIDS/HIV-1	Virus	Chimpanzee	ca. 1931 CE
AIDS/HIV-2	Virus	Monkey	Twentieth century

[a] This date (1492) represents the end of Spain's civil war against the Muslims in southern Spain. The thousands of non-combat deaths during 1489–90 among the Spanish soldiers seem likely to have been caused by the first outbreak of typhus in Europe.

CE = Christian Era; BCE = Before Christian Era.

Source: Weiss (2001).

Weiss 2001) lists some examples, showing probable animal source and date.

2.5.2 Second historical transition

When early Eurasian civilizations, increasingly large and powerful, came into military and commercial contact ca. 1500–3000 years ago, they inadvertently swapped their dominant infections. Thus, Rome, China, and the eastern Mediterranean exchanged their germ pools, often with catastrophic results—such as the Justinian Plague of AD 542 that devastated Constantinople and the Roman Empire. The historical record shows that China suffered a series of massive epidemics during these times (McNeill 1976).

This second great historical transition entailed a trans-Eurasian equilibration of infectious disease agents. There is evidence that European populations became increasingly adapted, genetically and culturally, to many of these now endemic or recurring infectious diseases. Presumably, the same was true at the eastern end of Eurasia, in the ancient vast civilization of China. Contact with the bubonic plague in Europe, however, had only been very occasional, and the disaster of the Black Death in vulnerable mid-fourteenth-century Europe came late in this second transitional period.

2.5.3 Third historical transition

The third transition resulted from European exploration and imperialism, beginning ca. AD 1500 and continuing over much of the past five centuries. This caused the trans-oceanic spread of often-lethal infectious diseases. The devastating impact of the repertoire of infections taken to the Americas by the Spanish conquistadors is well known. Without smallpox, Cortes may not have conquered the mighty empire of the Aztecs (Diamond 1997; Weiss 2001). Similar processes occurred with European explorations of the Asia-Pacific region, European settlement in Australia, and the trans-Atlantic slave trade.

An interesting sidelight on this third transition comes from Charles Darwin's two-month visit to eastern Australia in 1836, en route home after his stopover in the Galapagos islands. In his *Journal* (1839) Darwin writes, following his observations of diseases in Australian Aboriginals:

Besides these several evident causes of destruction, there appear to be some more mysterious agency generally at work. Wherever the European has trod, death seems to pursue the aboriginal. We may look to the wide extent of the Americas, Polynesia, the Cape of Good Hope, and Australia, and we shall find the same result.

Darwin later continues:

It is certainly a fact, which cannot be controverted, that most of the diseases that have raged in the islands during my residence there, have been introduced by ships; and what renders this fact remarkable is that there might be no appearance of the disease among the crew of the ship which conveyed this destructive importation.

Here, half a century before the elucidation of the germ theory, this great naturalist was (as ever) making incisive observation and inference.

2.5.4 Fourth historical transition

Today, we are living through the fourth great historical transition. This time, though, the scale is global and changes are occurring on many fronts. The contemporary spread and increased liability of various infectious diseases, both new and old, reflect the separate and combined impacts of widespread demographic, environmental, social, technological, and other rapid changes in human ecology. Global climate change, one of the greatest of the human-induced global environmental changes now underway, will also have diverse impacts upon the patterns of infectious disease occurrence.

The globalization of our economic activities and culture, the rapidity of distant contact, the spread and intensification of urbanization, and our increasing reliance on either intricate or massive technology, are reshaping the relations between humans and microbes. In particular, we are destabilizing ecosystems in ways that favour the proliferation of the *r* species—that is, those small opportunistic species that (in contrast to the larger *K* species such as ourselves) reproduce rapidly, invest in prodigious output rather than intensive parenting, and have mechanisms to efficiently disperse their offspring. Pathogens are typical

Table 2.2 Indicative relative importance of various categories of environmental and social influences on infectious disease emergence, in each of the four major historical transitions (see also commentary in text)

Category of influence	Historical transition			
	First (local: 5–10K years ago)	Second (continental 1–3K years ago)	Third (inter-continental 200–500 years ago)	Fourth (global current)
Changes in human–animal contacts	++++	+	+	++
Changes in social–demographic conditions	+++	++	++	+++
Environmental changes	++	+	+	++++
War, conquest	0	+++	++++	++
Trade, travel, population mobility	0	+++	+++	++++
New technologies (food production, healthcare, etc.)	+	0	0	++

r species, and they live today in a world of increasing opportunity.

Table 2.2 makes a notional comparison of the relative importance of major categories of environmental and social factors within each of the four historical transitions. (Note: the relativities are more meaningful within each of the four transitions, rather than between the transitions.) This necessarily inexact exercise underscores the changing configuration of social and environmental influences on infectious disease patterns. It also indicates that a more intensive set of influences applies in today's world.

2.6 Social and environmental influences on emerging infections: some examples

The following section provides some examples of emerging infectious diseases, considered under major categories of environmental and social influences, particularly patterns of travel, trade, and land use.

2.6.1 Travel and trade

Wherever we travel, unseen microbes accompany us. The plague bacterium, *Yersinia pestis*, accompanied Roman legions returning from the Middle East fifteen centuries ago. In mid-nineteenth-century London, John Snow noted that cholera epidemics followed major routes of commerce between Asia and Europe, appearing first at seaports when entering a new region. Today, however, the speed, volume, and reach of travel are unprecedented in human history, offering multiple potential routes for microbial spread around the globe.

The African malaria vector mosquito *Anopheles gambiae* gained entry to Brazil in 1937. Apparently, the mosquito migrated from western Africa on the mail-boats that traversed the Atlantic in 3–4 days. In the ensuing years, this mosquito species spread along the Brazilian coastal region and inland, and caused up to 50,000 deaths. (Subsequently, in the early 1940s, an extraordinarily intensive eradication campaign eliminated the mosquito.)

In today's globalizing economy, this story is often repeated. Dengue fever, which is numerically the most important vector-borne viral disease of humans, provides a good example. A major mosquito vector for the dengue fever virus, *Aedes albopictus* (the 'Asian tiger mosquito'), has spread widely in recent years via the unwitting intercontinental exportation of mosquito eggs in used car tyres into Africa and the Americas (Reiter and Sprenger 1987). Although dengue is primarily a tropical disease, its extension in recent decades into various temperate countries reflects both the introduction of the disease's main mosquito vector species, *Aedes aegypti* (which is behaviourally adaptable to a cold climate), and the increase in imported cases resulting from increased air travel (Kuno 1995).

This vector species, which breeds in water-containing sites typically found in the urban environment, has made extraordinary evolutionary adjustments to coexist with humans, having originated in forests of Africa. The vector has followed humankind on its travels and migrations around the world (Monath 1994).

Neisseria meningitidis, a global pathogen, causes seasonal epidemics of meningitis in parts of Africa: the so-called 'meningitis belt'. The disease has now spread more widely. Studies with molecular markers have shown that Muslim pilgrims brought an epidemic strain of *N. meningitidis* from southern Asia to Mecca in 1987, where they passed it on to pilgrims from sub-Saharan Africa who subsequently initiated, after returning home, strain-specific epidemic outbreaks in 1988 and 1989 (Moore *et al.* 1989).

The globalization of the food market has accentuated the movement of pathogens from one region to another. For example, the commercial movement of foods, particularly fruits and vegetables, also redistributes microbial resistance genes along with the microbes. For example, an outbreak of cholera in Maryland, USA, was traced to imported contaminated frozen coconut milk (Taylor *et al.* 1993). Alfalfa sprouts grown from contaminated seeds sent to a Dutch shipper caused outbreaks of infections with *Salmonella* species in both the United States and Finland (Mahon *et al.* 1997).

A primary drive that underlies migration is the urge to enter the cash economy, allied with the international demand for both skilled and unskilled workers in a globalizing marketplace. Rapid urbanization tends to boost old infectious diseases such as childhood pneumonia, diarrhoea, tuberculosis, and dengue. It also facilitates the spread of various 'emerging' diseases; for example, high-rise housing creates new risks—as recently observed for SARS in Hong Kong. Such housing also increases family breakdown, drug abuse, sexually transmitted infections, and HIV (Cohen 2003).

The disease West Nile virus, newly emergent in North America, further illustrates the impact of long-distance trade and travel. The disease originated in Africa, and occurs sporadically in the Middle East and parts of Europe. It was unknown in North America until it arrived in New York in 1999, via an infected mosquito on an aeroplane. Birds were affected first, humans later. There were apparently favourable conditions for the virus to survive and spread within New York City. They were:

1. Early season rain and summer drought provided ideal conditions for *Culex* mosquitoes.
2. July, 1999, was the hottest July on record for New York City.
3. Suburban/urban ecosystems support high numbers of select avian host and mosquito vector species adapted to those conditions, enabling close interaction of mosquitoes, birds, and humans.
4. High populations of susceptible bird species existed, especially crows.

West Nile virus then spread rapidly across the United States and by early 2004 had established itself as an endemic virus, harboured by animals including birds and horses and transmitted via mosquitoes. There was a sharp increase in the number of human cases, involving most US states, during 2002–3. In July 2003, Mexico declared a state of emergency when West Nile virus arrived in that country. There was concern that the disease could spread more rapidly in Central and South America than in North America because the warmer Latin American countries nurtured large bird populations and year-round mosquito populations.

2.6.2 Land use and environmental change

As Rene Dubos (1980) noted, humans have always changed their environments. We are, as ecologists say, 'patch disturbers'. The increasing scale of our intervention in the environment—both deliberately (e.g. land clearing, urbanization) and as collateral impact (e.g. global climate change, species extinctions)—is inevitably accelerating the rate of emergence of new infectious diseases. The main human-induced environmental changes that affect infectious disease risk include: tropical deforestation, road building, irrigation, dam building, local/regional weather anomalies, intensified crop and animal production systems, urban sprawl, continued poor sanitation, and pollution of coastal zones.

A Working Group on Land Use Change and Infectious Disease Emergence, comprising several dozen scientists from around the world, met in 2002 and ranked the various environmental factors associated with land-use according to their 'public health impact' on emerging diseases (Patz and Confalonieri 2004). The top 12 environmental changes, in descending order of impact, were:

1. Agricultural development;
2. Urbanization;
3. Deforestation;
4. Population movement;
5. Introduced species/pathogens;
6. Biodiversity loss;
7. Habitat fragmentation;
8. Water and air pollution (including via heightened respiratory susceptibility);
9. Road building;
10. Impacts of HIV/AIDS;
11. Climatic changes;
12. Hydrological changes, including dams

Many natural systems—forests, drylands, or cultivated systems—contain a distinct, exclusive, set of infectious diseases. However, several major diseases, including malaria and dengue, occur across many ecosystems. Malaria is transmitted by 26 different species of anopheline mosquitoes, each of them dominant in particular habitats and locations. Because each species responds differently to a specified land-use change, it is difficult to generalize the impact of ecosystem change effects across regions. Some other diseases such as yellow fever, however, can be transferred across ecosystems. The disease's natural, sylvatic, zoonotic cycle is between mosquitoes and monkeys high in forest canopies, but yellow fever can move into savannah, agricultural, and urban areas in the wake of activities such as logging or forest clearing.

2.7 Ecological disruptions

Various emerging infectious diseases can be considered in relation to the following six main types of ecological disruption, each of which entails a land-use component (Patz and Confalonieri 2004).

1. Altered habitat, with proliferation of reservoir or vector populations.
2. Biodiversity change and habitat fragmentation.
3. Ecosystem changes and loss of predators.
4. Intensified farming and animal husbandry.
5. Niche invasion.
6. Host transfer.

First, 'hantavirus pulmonary syndrome' provides an example of altered habitat, causing proliferation of reservoir or vector populations. Rodent-borne hantavirus occurs widely in agricultural systems, as in South America and east Asia, and in arid grasslands in North America and elsewhere. In mid-1993, an unexpected outbreak in humans occurred in the Four Corners region of southwest USA (Parmenter *et al.* 1993). The infection entailed acute respiratory distress, with high fatality. This 'hantavirus pulmonary syndrome' was traced to infection with a previously unrecognized virus, maintained primarily within the common native deer–mouse. Human infection occurs via contact with dried, wind-blown, excretions of infected mice. Apparently, the El Niño event of 1991–2, with its unseasonally heavy summer rains, hugely boosted the local rodent populations, and potentiated the 1993 outbreak (Glass *et al.* 1995; Engelthaler *et al.* 1999). Populations of deer–mice were 10–15-fold higher than during the previous 20-year seasonal average (Parmenter *et al.* 1993).

Second, biodiversity change and habitat fragmentation is well illustrated by the process of deforestation, with habitat fragmentation that increases the 'edge effect'—which promotes pathogen–vector–host interaction. This process has contributed, in recent decades, to the emergence of the various viral haemorrhagic fevers in South America. These viral infections are caused by arenaviruses that have wild rodents as their natural hosts. They have been described especially in Argentina (Junin virus), Bolivia (Machupo virus), and Venezuela (Guanarito virus) (Maiztegui 1975; Simpson 1978; Salas *et al.* 1991). These haemorrhagic fever infections typically occur in outbreaks ranging from a few dozen to thousands of cases. Outbreaks have mostly occurred in rural populations, when individuals become infected by contact with contaminated rodent excretions. The Machupo virus provides a good example. Forest clearance in Bolivia in the early 1960s, which was accompanied by blanket spraying of DDT to control malaria mosquitoes, led, respectively, to infestation of cropland by *Calomys* mice and to the poisoning of the rodents' usual predators (village cats). The consequent proliferation of mice and their viruses resulted in the appearance of a new viral fever, the Bolivian (Machupo) haemorrhagic fever, which killed around one-seventh of the local population.

Third, ecosystem changes may entail the loss of predator species, with resultant imbalance in the animal host species for a human pathogen. Lyme disease illustrates this category of ecologically disruptive factor. This bacterial disease was first identified in the northeast United States in 1976 in the town of Old Lyme. The ixodic ticks that transmit the spirochaete *Borrelia burgdorferi* normally feed on deer and white-footed mice, with the latter being the more competent viral host species. However, forest fragmentation has led to changes in biodiversity. This includes the loss of various predator species—wolves, foxes, raptors, and others—and a resultant shift of ticks from the less to the more competent host species (as white-footed mice have become relatively more numerous, because of the reduced 'dilution' effect of biodiversity). These changes, along with middle-class suburban sprawl into woodlands, have all been interconnected in the occurrence of this disease (Glass *et al.* 1995; Schmidt and Ostfeld 2001).

The fourth category, intensified farming and animal husbandry, is well illustrated by the apparent interactions between avian viruses and humans in rural south China and its environs. This interaction has been widely posited to underlie the emergence of new strains of influenza virus (perhaps with intervening passage through domesticated pigs). The influenza viruses are unstable genetically and are thus well adapted to evading host defences. Influenza viruses, when replicating in infected humans or animals, can undergo genetic rearrangement. This scrambling of genetic material, albeit usually minor, serves to ensure that animals and humans remain susceptible to at least some new strain of the virus during each subsequent season.

Niche invasion, the fifth category, occurs when a pathogen invades a new or recently vacated niche. A good example is the Nipah virus, which emerged as a cause for human disease in Malaysia in 1999, and resulted in over 100 deaths (Chua *et al.* 2000). This highly pathogenic virus emerged from its natural reservoir host species (fruit bats) via domestic animals (pigs) as amplifier hosts. The ecological trigger appears to have been a complex series of human alterations to fruit bat habitat and agriculture in combination with a period of drought (Daszak *et al.* 2001; Chua *et al.* 2002). Three considerations appear to be particularly relevant.

1. The virus does not appear to pass directly from bats to humans.
2. The fruit bat's habitat has been largely replaced in peninsular Malaysia by oil palm plantations.
3. Deforestation in adjacent Sumatra, coupled with a major El Niño-driven drought, led to significant seasonal air-pollution haze events that cover Malaysia. This reduced the flowering and fruiting of forest trees that are the natural food of fruit bats thus impairing their food supply.

Thus, the Nipah virus outbreak in 1999 was associated with a marked decline in forest fruit production. This caused the encroachment of fruit bats (the key Nipah virus reservoir) into pig farms, where fruit plantations were also maintained. Infected pigs then passed on the viral infection to pig farmers (Chua *et al.* 2002).

Finally, changes in ecological relations may result in host transfer, when a pathogen manages to cross the species barrier. In this important situation a genuinely new human infectious disease can arise.

The HIV/AIDS pandemic illustrates this perennial risk—we now know that SIV mutants passed into humans sometime during the twentieth century (see also Table 2.1). Bushmeat hunting in Africa has led to other local episodes of infectious disease emergence (Patz and Wolfe 2002): for example, forest workers cutting up chimpanzee meat have become infected with Ebola virus.

This cross-species transmission is, of course, bi-directional. That is, it can also entail non-human primate species and other valuable wildlife being infected with human pathogens. For example, the parasitic disease, Giardia, was introduced to the Ugandan mountain gorilla by humans through ecotourism and conservation activities (Nizeyi *et al.* 1999). Non-human primates have acquired measles from ecotourists (Wallis and Lee 1999).

2.8 Human-induced global climate change

Many pathogens and their vectors are very sensitive to climatic conditions, particularly temperature, surface water, and humidity. Over the past decade, it has become increasingly certain that humans not only face human-induced climate change (see Fig. 2.1), because of the continuing excessive emission of greenhouse gases, but that the process has indeed begun (IPCC 2001). A recent authoritative review paper states: 'Modern climate change is dominated by human influences, which are now large enough to exceed the bounds of natural variability' (Karl and Trenberth 2003).

The frequency and geographical range of some plant and animal infectious diseases have reportedly changed over recent years, at least partly in response to climate change (Harvell *et al.* 2002). For human infectious diseases, the causal configuration is intrinsically more complex (entailing many more demographic, social, and technological influences), and therefore it is more difficult to assess the contribution of recent climate change. Nevertheless, there is some suggestive evidence of an influence of recent climate change upon cholera outbreaks in Bangladesh (Rodo *et al.* 2002), an extension of tick-borne encephalitis in Sweden (Lindgren and Gustafson 2001) and, more

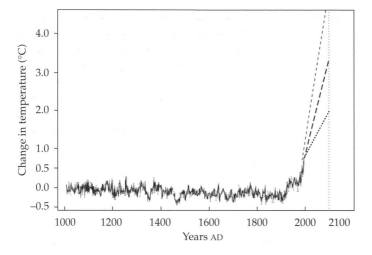

Figure 2.1 Reported variations in the Earth's average global surface temperature since AD 1000, supplemented by estimated range of increases over the coming century (IPPC 2001) in response to recent and ongoing build-up of atmospheric greenhouse gas concentration. Note also the rapid rise in temperature of ca. 0.4°C since 1975. Hatched lines show the range of plausible scenario-based globally averaged temperature increases estimated for the coming century by the IPCC (2001). The central estimate is for an approximately 3°C rise in temperature by 2100.

debatable, malaria occurrence in parts of eastern Africa (Patz *et al.* 2002).

The now-certain prospect of climate change raises the longer-term question as to how diseases such as malaria and dengue fever will respond over the coming century. Both statistical and biologically based ('process-based') models have been used, to assess how shifts in ranges of temperature and patterns of rainfall would affect the transmission potential of these diseases (Martens *et al.* 1999; Hales *et al.* 2002). Nevertheless, this genre of scenario-based modelling has not yet been able to address all aspects of the topic. For example, how will domestic and urban water use (particularly relevant to dengue fever transmission) change in a warmer world? Will climate change and associated ecosystem changes affect microbial mutation rates and successful speciation? How would an increase in the tempo of extreme weather events and natural disasters affect infectious disease occurrence? We still have many things to learn about how the impending shift to unfamiliar climatic conditions will affect the complex processes of infectious disease transmission, especially the vector-borne diseases.

2.9 Concluding comments

Over the last two centuries there have been accelerations in industrial and post-industrial changes in many aspects of human ecology, in population growth, and in the mobility of populations. In recent decades, various new infectious diseases have emerged, even as some pathogens that have been around for a long time were eradicated or rendered insignificant. Nature is always trying out new genetic variants; ecological niches open and close; human society's defences wax and wane. Environmental and ecological changes, economic and social changes, and international travel which drives a great movement of both pathogens and hosts, all affect the profile of infectious disease occurrence.

Assessing the relative importance of 'environmental' and 'social' factors in all of this is complex. The underlying initiating event, for a newly emergent disease, necessarily entails the entry into the human species, from an animal (broadly defined) source, of a normal zoonotic pathogen or of a fortuitous mutant pathogen. This event typically requires enhanced exposure of human subjects, and is best construed as an 'environmental' event. Such 'environmental' events, or encounters, have underlain the recent emergence of new infectious diseases such as HIV/AIDS, Lyme disease, the viral haemorrhagic fevers of South America, the Nipah virus and West Nile virus (within the United States). However, the particular environmental circumstance may be the result of some human behaviour or social practice, for example, migration into a new environment, land clearance, or climatic disturbance.

The subsequent dissemination of these newly evolving or newly discovered infectious diseases within human populations then depends on a mix of environmental and social factors. Malaria, tuberculosis, and dengue fever have all increased their compass over the past 20 years, particularly within poorer communities or groups (Fineberg and Wilson 1996; Farmer 1999). The disastrous spread of HIV/AIDS has had much to do with poverty, ignorance, prejudice, and inept government. Similarly, urbanization, long-distance travel, and freer sexual relations have all amplified the spread of many such diseases. Meanwhile, environmental mismanagement and change, whether in agricultural land-use, the damming of rivers, human-induced climate change, or evaporative air-conditioning, can all contribute to amplification of spread.

The experience of this past quarter century is obliging us to think more within an ecological framework. This accords with a view expressed by Edward Jenner just over two centuries ago. He stated: 'The deviation of man from the state in which he was originally placed by nature seems to have proved him a prolific source of diseases'.

We live in an increasingly globalized microbial world; a world that will inevitably continue to produce infectious disease surprises. We should therefore think, anticipate, and act more in terms of ecological balance, and less in terms of ambush, warfare, and arms race. Humans and microbes are not 'at war'. Rather, both parties are engaged in amoral, self-interested, coevolutionary struggle. We need to anticipate better the dynamics and consequences of that process. This has implications for environmental management, the alleviation of poverty as a generalized means of reducing susceptibility, the nurturing of social capital to ensure a stronger institutional base, the constraining of ecological folly arising from commercial pressures and excessive material consumption, and, of course, the restitution of society's public health capacities and function.

CHAPTER 3

Evolutionary genetics and the emergence of SARS Coronavirus

Edward C. Holmes and Andrew Rambaut

3.1 Summary

The recent appearance of severe acute respiratory syndrome coronavirus (SARS-CoV) highlights the threat to human health posed by emerging viruses. However, the key processes in the evolution of viral emergence are unclear, particularly whether emergence necessitates adaptation to the new host species. Herein we discuss the evolutionary genetics of viral emergence. We emphasize that although the high mutation rates of RNA viruses provide them with great adaptability, and explains why they are the main cause of emerging diseases, their limited genome size means that they are also subject to major evolutionary constraints. Understanding the mechanistic basis of these constraints is central in explaining why some RNA viruses are more able to cross species boundaries than others. Viral genetic factors have also been implicated in the emergence of SARS-CoV, with the suggestion that this virus is a recombinant between mammalian and avian coronaviruses. We argue, however, that the phylogenetic patterns cited as evidence for recombination are more likely due to variation in substitution rate among lineages, and that recombination is unlikely to explain the appearance of SARS in humans.

3.2 Introduction

Since the appearance of AIDS in the early 1980s, much has been written about the causes and consequences of emerging viral diseases. Yet despite increased disease surveillance, viral infections continue to appear in human and wildlife species.

There are 'new' viruses identified since the rise of AIDS, such as hepatitis C, Sin Nombre, Nipah, Hendra, and most recently SARS coronavirus. There are also more established pathogens, including West Nile virus and dengue virus, which have recently expanded their global prevalence. Even less progress has been made in what is perhaps the ultimate goal of research into emerging viruses—predicting what viruses are likely to affect human populations in the future.

Defining emerging viruses as those that have newly appeared or which have recently increased in prevalence and/or geographical range reveals some important general patterns. First, nearly all emerging viruses have RNA rather than DNA genomes. Although RNA viruses are ordinarily more commonplace than DNA viruses, this difference most likely reflects the differing evolutionary rates of these two types of infectious agent (see below). Second, nearly all emerging viruses have an animal reservoir, so that the process of viral emergence can usually be assigned to cross-species transmission (Cleaveland et al. 2001). For example, the human immunodeficiency virus type 1 (HIV-1), the major cause of AIDS, has its origins in the related simian immunodeficiency virus (SIV) found in chimpanzees (Gao et al. 1999), while SARS coronavirus (SARS-CoV) has close relatives in Himalayan palm civets (Guan et al. 2003), although it is not yet established that these are the source population for the human form of the virus. The most important exception to the rule that cross-species transmission is central to viral emergence is hepatitis C virus (HCV), which currently infects ~175 million people worldwide.

Despite surveying a number of animal species, the ultimate reservoir species for HCV remains a mystery. However, this is more likely to reflect the fact that the wrong species have been surveyed or the most closely related viruses are still too divergent in sequence to be recognized, than the complete absence of an animal reservoir altogether.

In many cases, the specific cause of emergence—why it has crossed from animals into humans—can be assigned to ecological factors, often relating to changes in land-use and deforestation (Morse 1995 and Chapter 2, this volume). Although a multitude of such ecological factors exist, they can often be placed into two general groups; changes in the proximity of the donor and recipient populations, so that humans have an increased chance of exposure to animal pathogens, and changes in the size and density of the donor and recipient populations, which increases both exposure and the likelihood that sustained networks of transmission will be established once a virus has entered a new species. Moreover, it is clear that as human ecology has changed through history with, for example, the rise of farming and later urbanization, so our burden of infectious disease has also increased (Dobson and Carper 1996). Although ecology seems to play the leading role in viral emergence, it is possible that genetic factors, in either the host or more probably the virus, also contribute to this process. As these genetic factors have only been considered in a cursory manner until now, we will outline in general terms the evolutionary genetic basis of viral emergence before considering the specific case of SARS coronavirus.

3.3 The evolutionary genetics of viral emergence

The elemental nature of the evolutionary interaction between host and virus is critical to understanding the process of emergence. On the host side, different species, or individuals within a species, may have differing susceptibilities to a specific virus infection. However, as host evolution obviously occurs at a much slower rate than virus evolution (Schliekelman *et al.* 2001), it is more

profitable to consider the differing abilities of viruses to jump species boundaries.

Perhaps the most fundamental question to address in this context is whether cross-species transmission and emergence requires adaptation to the new host species? In other words, how important is viral evolution in emergence? Under some models, a process of adaptation to the new host during the initial 'stuttering chains of transmission' is vital for the establishment of sustained transmission networks, as the basic reproductive rate of the virus (R_0) can be maximized at this stage (Antia *et al.* 2003). Alternatively, a virus may not be able to emerge in a new host unless the correct strain—one that will replicate and transmit in the recipient species (i.e. with R_0 already > 1)—is successfully transmitted, such that adaptation to the recipient species plays only a minor role. Although both models are likely to explain specific cases of emergence, there is perhaps more evidence for the latter. In particular, the far greater size of viral populations in the reservoir compared to the recipient species means that strains that may thrive in a new host are more likely to pre-exist in the former than evolve in the latter. Moreover, most emerging infections (in humans at least) are dead-end infections without subsequent transmission, indicating that any adaptation to the new host is usually unsuccessful (Woolhouse, personal communication). As an example, although avian influenza A viruses have successfully emerged and spread in human populations on three occasions during the twentieth century (in 1918, 1957, and 1968), most avian influenza viruses are unable to adapt to inter-human transmission. One of the most important characteristics in determining whether a virus will succeed in a new host is the ability to recognize the necessary cellular receptors (Baranowski *et al.* 2001). In the case of influenza A virus, this means a shift from binding to sialic acid receptors in a α2,3-linkage to galactose in birds, to a α2,6-linkage in humans. More generally, there is some evidence that the more conserved the cellular receptor in question, the more likely that cross-species transfer will occur (Woolhouse 2002).

If viruses do need to adapt to replicate in new host species, it follows that the more genetically variable the virus in question, then the more adaptable it will be. It is this fact that gives RNA viruses the edge in emergence (Woolhouse *et al.* 2001); the mutation rates of RNA viruses are usually many orders of magnitude greater than those of their DNA counterparts (although some populations of DNA viruses are highly variable which hints at higher mutation rates—Truyen *et al.* 1995; Sanz *et al.* 1999). On average, RNA polymerases generate an error in nearly every replication cycle (Drake *et al.* 1998; Malpica *et al.* 2002), so that when populations of RNA viruses are large, they will harbour a myriad of genetically different variants. Similarly, while many DNA viruses lead to persistent infections in their hosts, most RNA viruses (with the notable exception of retroviruses) only establish acute infections. This is critical to viral emergence because a short duration of infection means that the most likely way for RNA viruses to infect new host species is through cross-species transmission, rather than long-term co-speciation which is usually associated with persistence (Holmes 2004).

Although it is clear that the high mutation rates of RNA viruses enhance their adaptability, an unanswered question is whether all RNA viruses are equally equipped in this respect? Put another way, given an equivalent degree of exposure, are all RNA viruses equally likely to jump species boundaries? This question is at the heart of understanding the evolutionary basis to viral emergence, and although we are a long way from a complete answer, there is growing evidence that particular adaptive constraints make host switching more likely in some RNA viruses than others. An important (although largely untested) idea in this context is that there is a broad phylogenetic rule regarding the ability of a virus to jump hosts; the more phylogenetically distant the host species in question, the less likely that their viruses will be able to jump between them (DeFilippis and Villarreal 2000), again most likely reflecting differences in cell receptor usage. As a case in point, the reservoir populations for most human viruses are other mammalian species, and while we probably eat virally infected plant matter on a regular basis we do not suffer the viruses experienced by plants (Hull *et al.* 2000). On a more localized scale, studies of the human and simian

immunodeficiency viruses suggest that the ability of these viruses to jump species to some extent reflects the phylogenetic relationships of the hosts (Charleston and Robertson 2002), although that HIV-2 jumped from sooty mangabey monkeys to humans shows that exceptions are possible (Hahn *et al.* 2000). If true, such a phylogenetic trend corresponds to a simple evolutionary rule; the more a species is specialized to one environment, the less likely that it will be able to adapt to new environments (Bell 1997). The rapid pace of RNA virus evolution means that these host specificities are likely to be established quickly, as observed in experimental systems (Turner and Elena 2000). Testing the extent of the relationship between phylogenetic distance and the ability to jump hosts should be one of the key areas for future research into viral emergence.

At face value, it may seem strange that with their remarkable power of mutation RNA viruses are not able to exploit every adaptive solution. Ironically, the constraints faced by RNA viruses may themselves be a function of their high mutation rates, as this may limit their genome size which in turn hinders their ability to increase complexity. The causal link between mutation rate and genome size can be made by invoking the 'error threshold'. This theory was first introduced by Eigen (1987) as a crucial element in the evolution of the first RNA replicators, though in reality in can be extended to any living system (Maynard Smith and Szathmáry 1995). In simple terms, error threshold theory states that there is a maximum error rate that is tolerable for a genome of a particular size; as most mutations are deleterious, longer genomes than those imposed by the error threshold would see an over-burdening with deleterious mutations leading to dramatic fitness losses and eventual extinction. Hence, for RNA viruses that have high mutation rates because of their replication with intrinsically error-prone RNA polymerases, genome sizes must be small to prevent the accumulation of a deleterious mutation load.

Evidence for an error threshold in RNA virus evolution comes from a number of sources. First, RNA viruses occupy a very narrow range of genome sizes, with a median size of only ~9 kb and a maximum size of ~32 kb, as exhibited by some

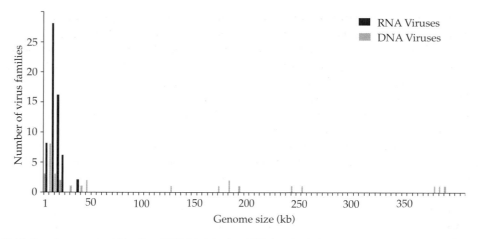

Figure 3.1 Distribution of genome sizes of families of RNA (black bars) and DNA (grey bars) viruses.
Source: www.ncbi.nlm.nih.gov/ICTV/.

coronaviruses. In contrast, DNA viruses range in size from a few thousand bases to almost 400 kb (Fig. 3.1), indicating that the upper limit on genome size cannot be due to common virological factors, such as capsid size or packaging requirements. Second, in experiments in which mutagens are applied to populations of RNA viruses as a form of antiviral therapy, thereby increasing the mutation rate, fitness declines dramatically. This suggests that the new mutation rate has breached the error threshold (Sierra *et al.* 2000; Crotty *et al.* 2001). Finally, there is a statistically significant negative correlation between nucleotide substitution rate (which reflects the background mutation rate if most mutations are neutral) and genome size, exactly as predicted under the error threshold model (Jenkins *et al.* 2002). The relationship between genome size and mutation rate is of particular importance for coronaviruses like SARS-CoV; as their genomes are relatively long, their mutation rates should be correspondingly low, which seems to be the case in at least some of the data sets analysed to date (Yeh *et al.* 2004).

By limiting genome size, high mutation rates constrain RNA virus evolution (Eigen 1996; Holmes 2003). In particular, small genome sizes mean that sequence regions may sometimes encode multiple functions and that individual mutations will be subject to rather complex fitness trade-offs. In short, pleiotropy and epistasis are expected to be common-place in RNA virus evolution.

Importantly, sequence analyses are starting to provide evidence for adaptive constraints in RNA virus evolution (some of which may also be found in small DNA viruses). For example, many RNA viruses utilize overlapping reading frames as this obviously increases the information content in small genomes. Similarly, because the limit to genome size means that relatively few nucleotide sites are free to vary, convergent evolution, in which the same solution evolves on multiple occasions, appears to be relatively common in RNA viruses (Cuevas *et al.* 2002). On a larger scale, there is growing evidence that intricate fitness trade-offs are important in shaping RNA virus evolution. A particularly powerful example concerns the arthropod viruses of vertebrates ('arboviruses'), which are unusual in that they replicate in hosts that are phylogenetically very different. From the argument presented earlier, such a life history strategy might be expected to be extremely difficult, given the very different nature of the host cells in each case. Analyses of selection pressures (Woelk and Holmes 2002) and substitution rates (Jenkins *et al.* 2002) have revealed that arboviruses are indeed subject to complex fitness trade-offs. Finally, the upper-limit on the genome sizes of RNA viruses means that they are less able to undergo gene duplication and lateral gene transfer (either from hosts or other viruses), evolutionary processes that appear to be common in the evolution of bacteria (Daubin *et al.* 2003), eukaryotes (McLysaght *et al.* 2002), and large DNA viruses (McLysagh *et al.* 2003). Interestingly, coronaviruses represent one of the few examples of lateral gene transfer in an RNA virus, as viruses assigned to the mammalian group 2 coronaviruses have seemingly acquired the haemagglutinin-esterase (HE) gene from influenza C virus (Marra *et al.* 2003).

Finally, it is a simple matter to predict that constraints to virus evolution in general will also affect their ability to emerge in new host species in particular. Hence, although all RNA viruses are likely to mutate rapidly, it is not necessarily the case that they will always be able to adapt to replicate and transmit in a new host species; the intricate epistatic and pleiotropic environments experienced by a particular virus may mean that the mutations required to infect a new host species will lower some other component of fitness, even if they are relatively simple to produce by mutation. As such, documenting the details of pleiotropy and epistasis in virus evolution is likely to be crucial to understanding their emergence.

3.4 What role has recombination played in the emergence of SARS coronavirus?

Apart from mutation, there is growing evidence that some RNA viruses are able to generate adaptively useful genotypic variation through recombination (Worobey and Holmes 1999). One such group is the coronaviruses, within which recombination in the spike glycoprotein has been extensively described (reviewed in Lai 1996). More controversially, it has also been suggested that SARS-CoV may be the result of a recombination of different coronavirus lineages (Rest and Mindell 2003; Stanhope *et al.* 2004; Stavrinides and Guttman 2004), an event that may have been central to its recent emergence in humans (Stanhope *et al.* 2004; Stavrinides and Guttman 2004). Although a variety of different recombination events have been proposed, they follow the same general scheme in which a mammalian coronavirus assigned to group 1 (such as human coronavirus 229E) or group 2 (such as mouse hepatitis virus) has recombined with an avian coronavirus assigned to

group 3 (such as infectious bronchitis virus), giving rise to the distinct evolutionary lineage represented by SARS-CoV. If true, this would represent one of the few documented cases in which a distinct genetic event has played a key role in viral emergence.

The claim that SARS-CoV has a recombinant history is based on the presence of phylogenetic incongruence; an observation that different gene regions give rise to phylogenetic trees with different topologies. Although incongruence is often a powerful signal for the action of recombination (reviewed in Posada *et al.* 2002), there are a number of reasons why the case for recombination in SARS-CoV should be questioned. First, SARS-CoV is clearly a distinct evolutionary lineage, approximately equidistant from the group 1, 2, and 3 coronaviruses, irrespective of what genes are analysed (Marra *et al.* 2003; Rota *et al.* 2003) (Fig. 3.2). Indeed, SARS-CoV is so phylogenetically distinct that it can be thought of as a fourth lineage of the coronaviruses. While this tree structure does not in itself rule out ancient recombination events among the different groups of coronaviruses, it means that recombination cannot have played a major role in the emergence of SARS-CoV in humans. This point is well illustrated by the phylogenetic position of the SARS-CoV strains from humans with respect to those isolated from the Himalayan palm civet. These viruses are almost indistinguishable at the amino acid level (and appear as almost identical in Fig. 3.2) and are much more closely related to each other in all gene regions than they are to the other groups of coronaviruses. If the civet is indeed the reservoir species for SARS-CoV, then the jump to humans occurred a very long time after any putative recombination events involving different coronavirus lineages.

It also seems likely that the main evidence for recombination—phylogenetic incongruence—is in reality caused by variation in evolutionary rate among lineages of coronaviruses. Coronavirus phylogenies are characterized by two patterns. First, sequences from different groups of coronaviruses are highly divergent, with average amino acid distances between them indicating that at least one amino acid replacement has been fixed at each site. Distances are even greater when the

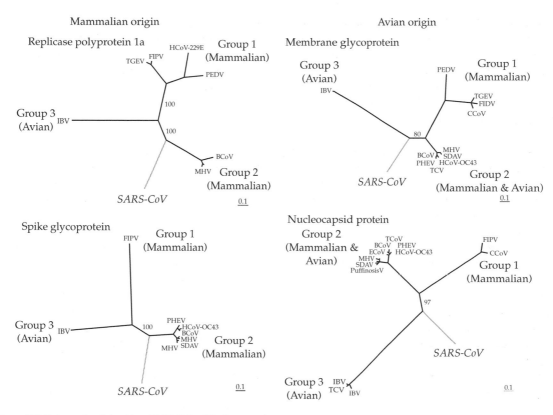

Figure 3.2 Phylogenetic relationships of SARS-CoV within the coronaviruses.

Notes: Phylogenetic trees were inferred using the maximum-likelihood option in TREE-PUZZLE (Strimmer and von Haeseler 1996) for the following gene regions and alignments kindly made available by Stavrinides and Guttman (2004): replicase polyprotein 1a (11 sequences, 338 amino acids), spike glycoprotein (12 sequences, 1270 amino acids), membrane glycoprotein (15 sequences, 214 amino acids), and nucleoprotein (17 sequences, 415 amino acids). In all cases the Whelan–Goldman model of amino acid replacement was used (Whelan and Goldman 2001). A gamma distribution of rate heterogeneity was also incorporated, with the value of the shape parameter (α) estimated from the empirical data (parameter values available from the authors on request). Numbers next to the main branches of the tree depict quartet puzzling support values, which give an indication of the reliability of each branch (with 100 signifying maximum support for the branch in question). All trees are unrooted, with branches drawn to a scale of the number of amino acid replacements per site. The following sequences were analysed (abbreviated viral names, where applicable, and NCBI accession numbers given in parentheses): group 1 coronaviruses: canaine coronavirus (CCoV; BAC65328, AAO33711), feline infectious peritonitis virus (FIPV; AAK09095, CAA29535, CAA39850, CAA39851), human coronavirus 229E (HCoV-229E; NP_073549), porcine epidemic diarrhoea virus (PEDV; AF353511), and transmissible gastroenteritis virus (TGEV; AJ271965); group 2 coronaviruses: bovine coronavirus (BCoV; AF220295, P26020), equine coronavirus (ECoV; AAG39339), human coronavirus OC43 (HCoV-OC43; P33469, Q01455, S44241), murine hepatitis virus (MHV; AF029248, AF201929, AF208066, CAA28484, NP_068668, P18446), porcine haemagglutinating encephalomyelitis virus (PHEV; AAL80031, AAM77004, AAM77005), puffinosis virus (CCAD67607), and rat sialodacryoadenitis coronavirus (SDAV; AAF97738, AAF97742); group 3 coronaviruses: infectious bronchitis virus (IBV; AAF35863, AAK83027, AJ311317) and turkey coronavirus (TCoV; P26021, AAF23872); SARS coronaviruses: Himalayan palm civet (SARS-CoV), strain SZ16 (AY304488) and human SARS coronavirus (SARS-CoV), strain CUHK-AG01 (AY345986).

arteriviruses (the closest known relatives of the coronaviruses) are included in the analysis as outgroups. Although using outgroups to root the tree of coronaviruses should, in theory, greatly assist in the analysis of recombination (Rest and Mindell 2003; Stavrinides and Guttman 2004), the sequences in this case are so divergent that accurate assessment of positional homology is extremely difficult, even with the most computationally powerful methods currently available. More importantly, even if there were no recombination events in the history of the three coronavirus lineages and SARS-CoV, by cutting up the genome into short fragments and estimating the phylogenetic relationships for each we would expect incongruence among the resulting phylogenies due to the stochastic nature of molecular evolution. This will be especially true in this case because the tree linking SARS-CoV to the other coronaviruses comprises variable length external branches (representing the four major lineages of coronaviruses), linked by a short internal branch (Fig. 3.2). Tree topologies with this general structure can be subject to a process of long branch attraction (Felsenstein 1978), in which the same changes evolve on unrelated long branches, such that rapidly evolving lineages tend to group together. Moreover, rate variation among lineages will also bias both network methods of phylogenetic inference such as split-decomposition (Worobey *et al.* 2002), which have been used to provide evidence for recombination in SARS-CoV (Stavrinides and Guttman 2004), and analyses of phylogenetic robustness such as the bootstrap or quartet puzzling.

To determine whether rate variation among lineages has produced a false-positive signal for recombination, we reanalysed the data provided in one of the papers suggesting that SARS-CoV has a recombinant history—that of Stavrinides and Guttman (2004). Using a variety of phylogenetic methods, these authors suggested that the replicase polyprotein 1a and the spike glycoprotein are of mammalian origin, since in trees of these proteins SARS-CoV is a sister-group to the group 2 coronaviruses, while the membrane glycoprotein and the nucleocapsid protein are of avian origin, as SARS-CoV is most closely related to the group 3 coronaviruses in these proteins. These conflicting phylogenetic positions are shown in Fig. 3.2. We performed a series of likelihood ratio tests to determine whether these four gene trees had significantly different tree topologies. Unlike the bootstrap or quartet puzzling, likelihood ratio tests are not biased by rate variation among lineages. We first constructed model tree topologies depicting each possible position of SARS-CoV, in which it was related, in turn, to coronavirus groups 1, 2, and 3. Next, the support for each competing tree was compared using a maximum likelihood method (full details are provided in the legend to Fig. 3.2). The results of this analysis are striking; in three of the four proteins analysed the likelihoods of the competing trees are so similar that none can be significantly favoured over any

other (Table 3.1). This strongly argues against the hypothesis of incongruence and hence recombination. In only a single comparison—that involving the highly variable spike glycoprotein—can one phylogenetic hypothesis, in this case that of SARS-CoV with the group 2 mammalian coronaviruses significantly reject the competing trees. Consequently, this analysis reveals that there is in reality little difference in the tree topologies inferred using the different genes of SARS-CoV, with any differences in branching order most likely reflecting rate variation among lineages. In short, localized differences in evolutionary rate among genes have produced tree topologies that show minor differences at their base, giving a false impression of ancient recombination. A similar lack of evidence for recombination in SARS coronavirus has independently been observed by other workers using phylogenetic methods (Gibbs *et al.* 2004).

Table 3.1 Maximum likelihood analysis of tree topologies depicting the possible phylogenetic positions of SARS-CoV within the coronaviruses

Protein/tree topology	$-Ln/L$[a]	Difference to ML tree	Significantly worse?
Membrane Glycoprotein			
SARS-CoV + group1	2727.04	2.91	No
SARS-CoV + group2	2725.69	1.56	No
SARS-CoV + group3	2724.13	ML tree	—
Nucleocapsid			
SARS-CoV + group1	5566.40	3.34	No
SARS-CoV + group2	5567.00	3.93	No
SARS-CoV + group3	5563.06	ML tree	—
Replicase Polyprotein 1a			
SARS-CoV + group1	4170.34	6.11	No
SARS-CoV + group2	4164.23	ML tree	—
SARS-CoV + group3	4171.44	7.21	No
Spike Glycoprotein			
SARS-CoV + group1	16,901.50	12.20	Yes
SARS-CoV + group2	16,889.30	ML tree	—
SARS-CoV + group3	16,901.89	12.60	Yes

[a] $-Ln/L = \log$ likelihood

Notes: Trees were compared using the Kishino–Hasegawa test (Kishino and Hasegawa 1989). In all cases, the competing topologies were compared to the maximum likelihood (ML) tree with $p < 0.05$ deemed as a significant difference. Only in the spike glycoprotein could one tree (SARS-CoV with the group 2 coronaviruses) be significantly favoured over another.

One way in which the problem of long branch attraction can be reduced is by including more taxa in the analysis, especially those that break-up long branches, as these tend to distribute convergent and parallel mutations more evenly across the tree, reducing their pulling power (Hillis 1996). Indeed, it is inevitable that the sample of coronaviruses available at present is only a small subset of those actually present in nature. With such a potentially small sample of lineages it is dangerous to make firm conclusions about the evolutionary history of SARS-CoV, particularly whether its ultimate ancestry lies with mammalian or avian coronaviruses. A key task for the future should therefore be a more extensive sampling of the phylogenetic diversity of coronaviruses in nature. However, on current data the evidence that SARS-CoV has a recombinant history is weak at best, and there is nothing to suggest that recombination has played a role in the emergence of SARS in humans.

3.5 Conclusions

Viral diseases pose a continual threat to human populations. As we live in ever larger populations and become increasingly mobile it is inevitable that new viruses, like SARS-CoV, will appear in the future. Although in most cases it is ecological changes that trigger viral emergence, as is probably the case with SARS, it is also evident that some viruses are better equipped to jump species barriers than others. The study of viral evolutionary genetics is therefore critical to understanding fundamental aspects of viral emergence. Genetics may also play a role in predicting what diseases might emerge in the future. In particular,

it will soon be possible to survey those animal populations that are most likely to harbour potentially emergent viruses. First, it is a relatively simple matter to make predictions about what sort of animals are most likely to carry viruses new to humans. As with humans, species with large and/or dense populations will carry a wide variety of pathogens as well as the most virulent diseases. This includes species of rodents, bats, and birds, and particularly those that live in close proximity to humans. A more significant advance is likely to come from molecular biology. It is now possible to develop degenerate PCR primers for families of RNA viruses (based on conserved viral genes) which can be used to survey animal populations, or even specific environments, for new viruses. These methods have already been used to survey microbial diversity in marine settings, uncovering a number of entirely new families of RNA viruses (Culley *et al.* 2003). More than simply surveying biodiversity, it may be possible to isolate any viruses detected in this manner and then determine whether they are able to grow in human cells. Although these techniques are only just beginning to be developed, and clearly represent a long-term research programme, they have the potential to provide efficient tools to survey the natural world for those pathogens that could have devastating effects on our health.

Acknowledgement

We thank the Wellcome Trust (grant 071979) and The Royal Society for financial support. Robin Weiss and Angela McLean gave extremely useful comments, while Mark Woolhouse and Rustom Antia provided informative discussion.

CHAPTER 4

Influenza as a model system for studying the cross-species transfer and evolution of the SARS coronavirus

Robin M. Bush

4.1 Summary

Severe acute respiratory syndrome coronavirus (SARS-CoV) moved into humans from a reservoir species and subsequently caused an epidemic in its new host. We know little about the processes that allowed the cross-species transfer of this previously unknown virus. I discuss what we have learned about the movement of viruses into humans from studies of influenza A, both how it crossed from birds to humans and how it subsequently evolved within the human population. Starting with a brief review of SARS to highlight the kinds of problems we face in learning about this viral disease, I then turn to influenza A, focusing on three topics. First, I present a reanalysis of data used to test the hypothesis that swine served as a 'mixing vessel' or intermediate host in the transmission of avian influenza to humans during the 1918 'Spanish flu' pandemic. Second, I review studies of archived viruses from the three recent influenza pandemics. Third, I discuss current limitations in using molecular data to study the evolution of infectious disease. Although influenza A and SARS-CoV differ in many ways, our knowledge of influenza A may provide important clues about what limits or favours cross-species transfers and subsequent epidemics of newly emerging pathogens.

4.2 The emergence of SARS coronavirus

Modern molecular and analytical tools allowed the rapid identification of SARS-CoV, a new member of the coronavirus family (Drosten *et al.* 2003; Ksiazek *et al.* 2003; Peiris *et al.* 2003*a*). Its genome was completely sequenced (Rota *et al.* 2003; Ruan *et al.* 2003) and the virus was confirmed as the cause of SARS (Fouchier *et al.* 2003) shortly after the onset of the epidemic. Sequence data were subsequently used to track the spread and evolution of the virus (Zhong *et al.* 2003; Guan *et al.* 2004; He *et al.* 2004; Yeh *et al.* 2004). Although it is as yet unclear exactly when cross-species transfer occurred, the first human cases known are from late autumn of 2002, just months before the major outbreak in May 2003. Thus we may have isolated SARS-CoV very soon after its initial transmission to humans. This should surely lead to better information on host source than we have obtained for influenza A, where we are limited to the study of a few poorly preserved samples from past decades. Nonetheless, we as yet do not know where SARS-CoV came from. Following up on reports that early cases of SARS occurred in animal handlers in the live markets of Guangdong Province, China, it was found that viruses very similar to human SARS-CoV could be isolated from masked palm civets (Paguma larvata) and raccoon dogs (Nyctereutes procyonoides), small rodent-eating mammals native to Southeast Asia (Guan *et al.* 2003). This suggests that these animals served as intermediate hosts between a natural reservoir species and humans. However, efforts to isolate SARS-CoV from these species outside the live markets have failed. SARS-CoV is relatively promiscuous: it has been shown to infect a wide range of mammals in the laboratory, including ferrets, domestic cats (Martina *et al.* 2003), and cynomolgus macaques (Rimmelzwaan *et al.* 2003). Thus the native host of SARS-CoV could be an unknown species that infected civets and other exotic food animals in their native habitat, on farms or en route to market. Rats have been suggested as agents of spread within the Amoy Hotel in Hong Kong, the primary epicentre of global spread (Ng 2003). Rodents might thus provide a common currency between the various types of small rodent-eating mammals found to harbour SARS-CoV in the markets. Unfortunately, as yet very little information is available on the occurrence of SARS-CoV in rodents in affected areas. Despite the lack of definitive evidence that civets outside the market system pose a threat to human health, massive and controversial extermination campaigns against civets have subsequently been carried out. In part, this may have been inspired by the initially successful attempt to rid the Hong Kong markets of avian influenza in 1997. These avian influenza A subtype H5N1 viruses infected at least 18 humans, 6 of whom died (de Jong *et al.* 1997; Claas *et al.* 1998; Subbarao *et al.* 1998). The H5N1 avian influenza A viruses responsible for the 1997 Hong Kong outbreak were unlike any known avian viruses. They appear, based on sequence data, to be reassortants between viruses from geese and viruses from either quail or teal (Guan *et al.* 1999; Hoffmann *et al.* 2000). These species are often caged in close proximity in live markets. Influenza viruses have a segmented genome and so are capable of forming reassortant progeny if two viruses infect a single host cell. Unfortunately, repeated culling measures have failed to contain the problem permanently, and H5N1 viruses are currently causing a devastating pandemic in domestic fowl across Southeast Asia. Many humans coming in contact with these birds have contracted the virus; in some cases they have died. Fortunately, there is thus far no evidence that the H5N1 virus has become adapted for transmission between humans. Nonetheless, this outbreak is of great concern because the vast number of infections increases the probability of avian–human reassortment.

4.3 The origin of influenza A

One of the most interesting aspects of the 1997 H5N1 outbreak in Hong Kong is that prior to that time direct transmission of avian viruses to humans had been reported rarely and was believed to be highly restricted. Influenza viruses from humans and birds are known to bind preferentially to different forms of the sialic-acid receptor on host cells. This preferential binding was thought to be the primary barrier against human infection by avian strains and led to the idea that swine, whose cells possess both the receptors preferred by avian and human influenza viruses, serve as intermediate hosts or 'mixing vessels' for the transmission of avian viruses to humans (Scholtissek 1990). This hypothesis is consistent with the observation that a massive outbreak of respiratory disease in swine occurred concurrently with the 1918 influenza pandemic in humans, and would explain why many epidemics and pandemics appear to originate in Southeast Asia, where agricultural practices put ducks, swine, and humans in close contact, as reviewed by de Jong *et al.* (2000). Swine can clearly be infected by both human- and avian-adapted influenza viruses. However, the role of swine in the cross-species transfer of influenza A to humans is, despite much study, still unclear. Here, I review two types of molecular analysis that have been used to try to determine the source of pandemic influenza viruses and the mechanisms by which they crossed species barriers. Both are, or probably will be, applied to the study of SARS; thus, I point out in some detail the limitations of these methods as well as what insight they can offer. At the end I review more general limitations in using molecular data to study the evolution of infectious disease.

4.4 Retrospective analyses based on phylogenetics

One method for dating prior events is to use molecular data to estimate current rates of genetic change, and then extrapolate backwards in time to the period of interest. This method was used to test the hypothesis that swine served as a

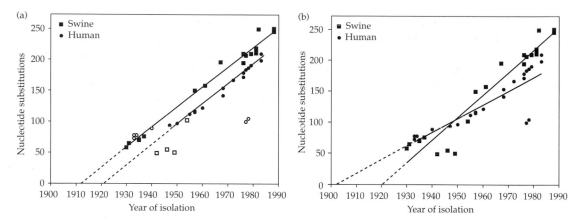

Figure 4.1 Cross-species transmission estimates for human and swine influenza A subtype H1N1. Genetic distances are measured from the root of a phylogenetic tree (not shown). Data from Scholtissek *et al.* (1993*a*,*b*). Rates of evolution for swine (squares) and human (circles) lineages are calculated as the slopes of the respective regression lines. Units are nucleotide substitutions per year. Extrapolation backwards in time (dashed lines) was used to determine the date of the initial transmission of the virus into these hosts. (a) Rates estimated using only the closed symbols, as in Scholtissek *et al.* (1993*b*). (b) Rates estimated using the complete dataset.

'mixing vessel' for the reassortment of avian and human-adapted influenza viruses in the origin of the 1918 'Spanish flu' pandemic (Scholtissek 1990). Scholtissek *et al.* (1993*b*) constructed a phylogenetic tree using sequence data for the nucleoprotein genes of 23 human and 24 swine influenza viruses. They calculated the genetic distance from the root of the tree to each isolate, then regressed distance against isolation date to estimate an average rate of evolution in nucleotide substitutions per year. The resulting plot is redrawn in Fig. 4.1(a). Assuming constant rates of evolution over time, they extrapolated backwards on the time (horizontal) axis to estimate when the original viruses were first transmitted to these new hosts. An estimate of the time of divergence from a common ancestor could have been obtained, had the lines not been parallel, from the point in time at which the lines crossed. Figure 4.1(a) shows the swine lineage intercepting the time axis around 1912, slightly before the human lineage, which intercepts the line at around 1920. However, the authors noted that if they had displaced the root of the tree (which appears to have been rooted at the midpoint) 12 nucleotide substitutions nearer to the swine lineage, the human and swine influenza lineages would have both crossed the time axis at around 1918. Although the authors offer no definitive conclusions as to which new host was

infected first, this analysis has often been used to suggest that an avian influenza virus was first transmitted to pigs and subsequently evolved the ability to infect humans around the time of the 1918 pandemic (Scholtissek *et al.* 1998; Webster 1998). However, it is possible to move the root of a tree arbitrarily in any number of directions. In this example, moving the root across the possible rooting options (from the base of the swine clade to the base of the human clade) produces widely varying and contradictory conclusions. If the tree was rooted at the base of the human clade, it would appear that the virus first infected humans in 1899 and then swine 35 years later, in 1934. If the tree was rooted at the base of the swine clade, it would appear that the virus first infected swine in 1891 and then humans in 1942, 51 years later. Obviously these rooting decisions should not be made arbitrarily. An outgroup should be used to root a tree if one is available. Adding A/Equine/Prague/56 (Reid *et al.* 2003) to the analysis shown in Fig. 4.1(a) suggests that the root should be moved four nucleotide substitutions closer to the swine lineage. Doing so suggests transmission to humans in 1900 and to swine in 1922, dates that are inconsistent with observed disease incidence. The use of a different outgroup sequence could well give different results. Unfortunately, for many groups of organisms the outgroup is unknown or may be only distantly related to the lineages of interest. This point is especially germane to the study of SARS-CoV because determining its nearest relative has proved problematic (Drosten *et al.* 2003; Eickmann *et al.* 2003; Marra *et al.* 2003; Rota *et al.* 2003) and may never be resolved. Another major limitation to these types of regression analyses is that they are very sensitive to the particular dataset used, especially when sample sizes are small. In this example, Scholtissek *et al.* (1993*b*) employed only 77% of the data points used to construct the phylogeny when estimating the regression lines in Fig. 4.1(a). The stated exclusion criterion was that the excluded points lay too far from the regression lines (Scholtissek *et al.* 1993*a*); the criteria for establishing those lines in the first place were not provided. Figure 4.1(b) shows the resulting plot had all data points been included. These results suggest that transmission to humans occurred in 1904 and to swine in 1921 (Fig. 4.1(b)). Neither of these dates are consistent with historical observations of disease incidence. In addition, the two regression lines diverge rather than converge as they approach the time axis. This gives the impression that these lineages did not diverge from a common ancestor; however, both are believed to have originated from avian strains (Reid *et al.* 2003). Clearly, this dataset would have provided no support for the 'mixing vessel' hypothesis if all the data used to construct the phylogeny had also been used in the regression analysis. There is always a risk in drawing conclusions from extrapolation of a regression analysis (Kuo 2002). In the case of emerging infectious disease, this technique is especially suspect because extrapolation relies on the assumption of a constant rate of evolution over time. The 1918 pandemic infected humans in waves of increasing severity in 1918 and 1919 before evolving into the (relatively) benign form we experience today. To assume a constant rate of evolution over this entire period is questionable. As noted by Cox *et al.* (1993) the influenza literature reports substantial variation in the rates of evolution for the different strains, even during very recent periods of time when the initial adaptation to humans is presumably over. One major cause of this variation is lack of data, another is drawing conclusions using data that cover only short periods of time. An illustration of rate variation for influenza A subtype H3N2 is shown in Fig. 4.2(a). Varying estimates of evolutionary rates have already been reported for SARS-CoV (I Ie *et al.* 2004; Yeh *et al.* 2004) despite the very short period of time it has been under study. Based on our experience with influenza, these estimates will change not only over time, if the virus continues to circulate, but also with the addition of more data for the time periods already studied.

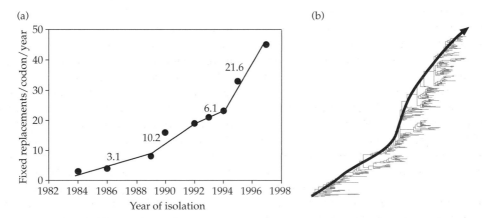

Figure 4.2 Variation over time in the rate of influenza A subtype H3N2 evolution. (a) Circles show the cumulative number of amino acid replacements fixed along the trunk of the tree (see arrow in (b); data from Bush *et al.* (1999)). The numbers indicate rates per year calculated over arbitrarily chosen short intervals of time as indicated by regression lines. Choosing different intervals would result in vastly different rate estimates.

4.5 Analysis of archived influenza viruses

The origins of pandemic influenza have also been examined through the study of archived viruses. The pandemics of 1957 and 1968 were clearly caused by reassortant viruses containing human and avian influenza genes. The influenza A genome is composed of eight segments, each containing one or two of its 11 genes. Influenza strains are typically referred to by the genetic variants of their surface proteins, haemagglutinin and neuraminidase. At present 15 haemagglutinin alleles (numbered H1–H15) and nine neuraminidase alleles (N1–N9) are known from waterfowl. These avian viruses are thought to be the ancestors of strains currently circulating in swine, horses, and humans (Webster et al. 1992). The 1918 pandemic strain carried H1 and N1 alleles. A descendant of this strain appears to have gained avian derived genes for surface proteins H2 and N2, and for PB1, one of the influenza polymerase genes, through reassortment in 1957. The resulting H2N2 strain circulated in humans until 1968 when it was replaced by a reassortant containing new avian H3 and PB1 genes (Scholtissek et al. 1978; Kawaoka et al. 1989). The resulting H3N2 virus continues to circulate in humans today. Although these reassortment events may have taken place within swine, there is no evidence to support this thesis from the sequence data, which implicate only avian and human sources. The origin of the deadly 1918 pandemic is less clear than those of the 1957 and 1968 pandemics. Ongoing studies of H1N1 influenza A viruses preserved in the archived lung tissue of two army soldiers and from an Alaskan Inuit woman frozen in permafrost, all victims of the 1918 pandemic, have yet to reveal why this strain was so deadly or exactly where it came from (Taubenberger et al. 1997; Reid et al. 1999). The haemagglutinin and neuraminidase alleles resemble the oldest available classical H1N1 swine influenza strains (from 1930), but share characteristics with modern avian H1N1 strains as well. Sequencing viruses isolated from waterfowl collected in 1917 and preserved in alcohol in the American Museum of Natural History has done little to resolve this mystery (Fanning et al. 2002;

Reid et al. 2003). An additional line of inquiry stems from X-ray crystallographic studies of haemagglutinin proteins reconstructed from 1918 sequence data. These data suggest that the binding site of the 1918 human virus is more avian-like than that of later H1N1 viruses (Gamblin et al. 2004; Stevens et al. 2004). But, as Reid et al. (2003) concluded, it appears, based on current material, that, if the 1918 human pandemic strain was avian-derived, it must have evolved undetected in a non-avian host for some time prior to the 1918 human pandemic. We have some knowledge of the molecular basis of host specificity for influenza viruses, such as the presence or absence of a sequence of basic amino acids at the haemagglutinin cleavage site, and a preferential binding to the α2,3-linked galactosidase found in birds rather than the α2,6-linked galactosidase found on human lung cells (reviewed by Zambon 2004). However, binding studies clearly showed these differences to be preferences rather than absolute barriers to infection (Matrosovich et al. 1993). This result is sadly supported by the many recent infections of humans with entirely avian viruses. Although it has long been known that sporadic infections of humans by avian viruses can occur (Shortridge 1992), transmission within the new host population is rare. Efficient transmission seemingly depends on a number of variables, and may well require that interacting coadapted sets of genes remain together through reassortment events (Rott 1992). New experiments using reverse genetics to construct influenza viruses with various combinations of human and avian genes will hopefully provide greater insight into the genetics of host specificity and modes of transmission. (Neumann et al. 2003). Evidence for direct infection of humans by avian viruses does not prove that swine have never been involved in the transmission of avian influenza to humans. It suggests, however, the existence of additional barriers to establishment in mammals. One barrier may be the lack of efficient transmission between individuals in the new host species. Birds generally harbour influenza viruses in their intestinal tract, not in their lungs. Thus avian viruses must adapt both to conditions in the mammalian respiratory tract and to airborne transmission. Dehydration during aerosol transmission among humans, for example, is a challenge not experienced during spread in faeces or in the aquatic environments of waterfowl. Differences in temperature and pH may also play a role. The genetics of transmission is clearly an area in need of study, but by its nature it is an impossible problem to address using humans. Although cynomolgus macaques infected with avian H5N1 influenza A produced a necrotizing pneumonia similar to that seen in the human fatalities of H5N1 infection (Rimmelzwaan *et al.* 2003), studying transmission using these animals is formidably expensive and in some eyes unethical, and, in addition, there is no guarantee that the results would be applicable to humans. Transmission studies of SARS-CoV in animal models might be similarly expensive and difficult to interpret.

4.6 Limitations of molecular data

The existing influenza sequence data are among the best available for studying the evolution of infectious disease. However, there are problems with using these data to study influenza evolution and population biology, and these limitations may hold true for SARS-CoV as well. One problem is the presence of laboratory artefacts in the sequence data. Although cell culture is increasingly used, amplification of the influenza virus by passage in embryonated hens' eggs has been standard laboratory practice for the culture of influenza viruses for many years. Egg passage is still required for strains that will be used in the influenza vaccine in the United States. Unfortunately, the haemagglutinin of human influenza viruses evolves rapidly to adapt to replication in eggs (Robertson 1993). The resulting sequences may thus contain replacements that either were not present or were at low frequency in the original viral sample. These laboratory artefacts often occur at sites involved in adaptation to humans as well as to eggs (Cox and Bender 1995). It is possible to estimate the proportion of amino acid replacements resulting from egg passage by comparing the numbers of replacements found in sequences in cell-passaged and egg-passaged isolates (Bush *et al.* 2000, 2001). In the HA1 domain of influenza A subtype H3N2 haemagglutinin, egg passage was associated with about 8% of amino acid replacements (Bush *et al.* 1999). Unfortunately, in the absence of controls—viruses that have never been passaged—it is impossible to determine which replacements in a dataset are artefacts. These artefacts inflate the amount of evolutionary change that one infers from sequence data. Because these artefacts are non-synonymous as opposed to synonymous substitutions, care must be taken to eliminate them from analyses seeking evidence of positive selection by the human immune system. One way to minimize such error is to discard changes assigned to the terminal branches of the trees when estimating substitution rates (Bush *et al.* 1999). Studies of positive selection in influenza that fail to exclude replacements selected for during egg passage routinely find evidence for selection on codons for which there is no evidence of a selective advantage in humans (Yang 2000; Yang *et al.* 2000; Huelsenbeck *et al.* 2001; Nielsen and Huelsenbeck 2002). In studies of positive selection thus far in SARS-CoV, some groups deleted possible artefacts (Ruan *et al.* 2003; He *et al.* 2004), while Yeh *et al.* (2004), after contrasting a direct polymerase chain reaction (PCR) product with sequences from isolates cultured in monkey kidney cells, did not find culture-induced artefacts to be a problem. These studies have so far found variable evidence for positive selection in SARS-CoV, which is not surprising given how few data are as yet available. Another difficulty in the molecular analysis of sequence data collected during disease surveillance is sampling bias. The World Health Organization (WHO) influenza surveillance system is purposefully biased towards sequencing viruses that differ antigenically from commonly sampled strains on the basis of the haemagglutination inhibition test. This bias causes an overestimation of positive selection on the haemagglutinin gene because only non-synonymous substitutions produce antigenic change. The WHO is the main source of influenza sequence data; thus this sampling bias is reflected in the composition of sequences present in Gen-Bank. Assuming that the frequencies of various genetic groups in GenBank reflect their frequencies in nature (Plotkin *et al.* 2002) will invariably lead to erroneous results under current WHO sampling protocols. Last, it can be very difficult to make accurate inferences about evolutionary relationships between distantly related organisms because of the resulting sequence dissimilarity. Conclusions may vary dramatically depending on how these sequences are aligned. Early reports that some genes in the SARS-CoV genome are the result of recombination (Rest and Mindell 2003; Stavrinides and Guttman 2004) may be alignment dependent. They may also share characteristics with a study claiming that the 1918 influenza haemagglutinin gene was a recombinant (Gibbs *et al.* 2001). This study has been criticized for not being robust with respect to the method of phylogenetic reconstruction (Worobey *et al.* 2002). Ideas about the recombinant origin of SARS-CoV as discussed in Chapter 3 of this volume may well change further as more data become available.

4.7 Suggestions for future research

The extent of the spread of most infectious diseases are vastly understudied in part because there is almost no emphasis on determining the occurrence of subclinical disease. Farmers in Southeast Asia have long been reported to carry antibodies to a number of avian influenza subtypes not known to circulate in humans, including the *H*5 allele, which was recently involved in outbreaks of human illness in Hong Kong (Shortridge 1992). Sera from healthy blood donors in Hong Kong contained antibodies to the H9N2 virus, suggesting prior infection by this strain (Peiris *et al.* 1999). Early serological reports suggested a subclinical infection rate with SARS-CoV of 13% in

animal traders (CDC 2003); however, as we learn more about the serological cross-reactivity of SARS-CoV with common coronaviruses such values may change. Surveillance rarely targets healthy people or geographical locations not experiencing a high incidence of disease. This may be why we are so often surprised by new outbreaks of infectious disease. We may also continue to be surprised if we expect new epidemics to arise from viruses that evolve from the most recently circulating strains. This is not always the case: in many instances new influenza-epidemic strains are descendants of viruses from years past, viruses that had persisted at low frequency while other strains caused our yearly epidemics (Cox *et al.* 1993). Because extensive surveillance for influenza has been in place for over 50 years, the influenza surveillance community is often aware of these lurking threats. Unfortunately, global surveillance does not exist for most known pathogens and is certainly lacking for those viruses, like SARS-CoV, that have yet to emerge from their even more poorly known animal hosts. Funding for such efforts is discussed in the heat of an outbreak; however, effective surveillance, even of human infectious diseases, is a long way from becoming a reality. Even less interest and money is being directed towards conservation of museum and medical archives, which as discussed in Section 4.4 have contributed much of what we know about the origin of pandemic influenza. One wonders whether tissue samples are being saved from the masked palm civets currently being destroyed in China: we may be in the process of burning the evidence.

CHAPTER 5

Management and prevention of SARS in China

Nanshan Zhong and Guangqiao Zeng

5.1 Summary

This chapter describes three different severe acute respiratory syndrome (SARS) events that took place in Mainland China between November 2002 and April 2004. The first confirmed case of SARS is now known to have presented in November 2002. A 43-year-old man who had eaten a meal of 'wild cat', presented with fever and diarrhoea a week later. He proved to be the harbinger of a major SARS epidemic in Guangdong Province in which 1512 people were infected and 58 died. The second event described here is a series of 4 cases that occurred between December 2003 and January 2004. Through lessons learned in the 2003 epidemic, these cases were successfully contained and no further cases of community acquired SARS were seen between January 2003 and the summer of 2004 when this text went to press. There were, however, two cases of laboratory acquired infections and secondary transmissions. The description of these forms the third SARS event described here.

5.2 The first Guangdong epidemic

The first case of SARS that I encountered at Guangzhou was a 41-year-old man who developed a high fever (39.6°C), malaise, myalgia for 3 days, bilateral infiltration in a chest radiograph, and no response to antibiotics (azithromycin and ofloxacin) (Xiao *et al.* 2003). The patient was referred to my institute (Guangzhou Institute of Respiratory Diseases) on 22 December 2002. On 27 December 2002, he developed severe hypoxaemia, presenting with tachypnoea (55 times per min) and poor oxygen saturation (oxygen index 137),

and was then intubated for mechanical ventilation. Methylprednisolone at a daily dose of 160 mg was given. After 34 days' ventilation, he was extubated and was discharged on 15 March 2003. During his admission we were told that another eight persons with a close contact history with him developed a similar pneumonia 8–10 days after his admission. At that time we had no idea what the diagnosis of the disease was and could only name it first as 'pneumonia with an unknown cause', then as 'atypical pneumonia'. At the end of March 2003 the patient was diagnosed as having SARS by a fourfold rise in serum SARS-CoV IgG antibody. Actually from a retrospective study in Foshan, it was confirmed that the first onset of SARS was on 16 November 2002, when a 43-year-old man presented with fever and diarrhoea after having an exotic meal ('wild cat') one week before (Zhou *et al.* 2003). The clinical picture and disease process of this Foshan case resembled the case mentioned above. No antibiotics helped his condition, and a cluster of cases among households and healthcare workers after an incubation period of 10 days or so was also noticed. When these cases were retrospectively analysed with ELISA tests in May 2003, the diagnosis of an early cluster of SARS cases was confirmed. After the first report of SARS at the end of December 2003, reports of SARS cases increased, first in the cities of Guangdong, then in Hong Kong, and then in other cities in Mainland China. The epidemic of SARS in Hong Kong began with the visit of an infected physician from Guangzhou in mid-February 2003 (Zhong *et al.* 2003). At least 16 visitors and guests at the index hotel where he stayed came down with the illness. These infected individuals in turn spread the disease to other cities including Toronto, Singapore, and Hanoi (Hsu *et al.* 2003; Poutanen *et al.* 2003) and subsequently to more than 30 countries and regions across five continents.

From the clinical epidemiology perspective, it was proved that the SARS epidemic originated from Guangdong (Chan-Yeung *et al.* 2003). Virus epidemiology also confirmed that SARS-CoV isolates from Guangzhou shared the same origin with those in other countries and had a phylogenetic pathway that matched the spread of SARS to other regions of the world (Zhou *et al.* 2003).

During the 2002–3 SARS epidemic in Guangdong, 1512 people were infected and 58 deaths occurred, with a case fatality rate of 3.8%, which ranked as the lowest in the world. In addition to the difference in the severity of the epidemic and age distribution among different countries or regions, rational management contributed partly to the low mortality in Guangdong. In those with critical SARS (rapid development of dyspnoea with a respiratory rate more than 30 times per minute, persistent high fever for more than 3 days, or rapid deterioration of the chest film with increased infiltrates progressing to a critical condition), use of corticosteroid (methylprednisolone 1–2 mg/kg/d) demonstrated a definite efficacy in 53% of patients. The Guangzhou experience showed that the percentage of bone necrosis (femur and knee) after corticosteroid therapy was 4%, which may be related to the steroid dosage; 20–30% of patients with critical SARS received non-invasive facial/nasal mask ventilation (mainly continuous positive airway pressure, CPAP), which enabled improvement of oxygenation in early stage and avoided the necessity for intubation. Data showed that non-invasive ventilation did not cause cross-infection (Zhong and Zeng 2003). The integration of traditional Chinese medicine and Western medicine further relieved dyspnoea and malaise and facilitated the resolution of pulmonary infiltration.

5.3 The last community-acquired infections

There were two events of SARS in Mainland China following the first outbreak.

The first consisted of four new cases of SARS that occurred from the end of December 2003 to January 2004 in Guangzhou. There was a close linkage of SARS-CoV between humans and small wild mammals, in particular civet cats, based on the following.

1. SARS-CoV (isolated or PCR (polymerase chain reaction)-tested) found in throat swab (faeces) specimens in 76% of civet cats being surveyed in Guangdong.
2. Serum SARS-CoV IgG was found in 40% of wild animal traders, which was much higher than in those with other occupations such as vegetable traders, butchers, and healthy individuals.
3. A high homology of the *S*-gene sequence of SARS-CoV isolated from throat swab specimens between the first case of SARS and the civet cat.
4. The second new case of SARS was a waitress working at a game food restaurant, where SARS-CoV-positive specimens (RT–PCR *N* and *M* genes) were found in five out of seven cages of civet cats.

It was thus highly suspected that civet cats were an important potential source of infection.

Civet cats are members of cat-like animals belonging to a large group of nocturnal mammals which are not true cats, although they look like cats. Along with other small mammals such as raccoon-dogs and ferret badgers, they possibly became infected from another, as yet unknown animal source, which is in fact the true reservoir of SARS in nature. However, by entering exotic food markets, these animals have become the topmost known link in the SARS transmission route. As such they represent a dangerous source of possible new infections that could undermine the prevention of SARS (Fig. 5.1). As game foods are considered to 'enhance the vitality of the body', the Cantonese consume them as tonics in substantial amount in the cold weather, and wildlife markets in Guangzhou blossom in winter each year. Given the poor management, open-air laying-out of traded animals, and cluttered sanitation in many wet markets, cross-infection, interspecies transmission, amplification, genetic convergence, and mixing of coronavirus are conceivably taking place. Animal traders standing in close proximity with these infected animals may be affected. This may be true for food processors

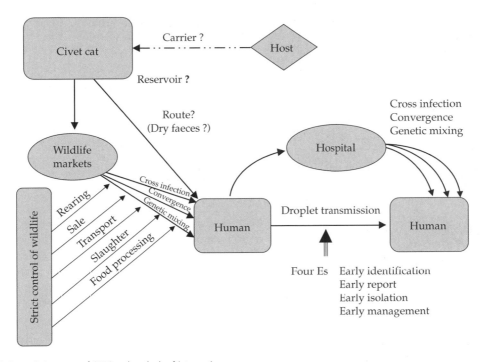

Figure 5.1 Transmission route of SARS and methods of intervention.

who slaughter infected animals in restaurant kitchens, causing SARS-CoV to spread from wildlife to humans, and thereby from human to human principally by droplet transmission.

At the beginning of 2004, the Guangdong local government and Department of Public Health had taken strong actions regarding: (1) strict control of the wildlife market, including a ban on rearing, sales, transport, slaughter, and food processing of small wild mammals and civet cats in particular. Seventeen rearing farms were closed within 5 days; (2) 'four earliness' (early identification, early report, early isolation, and early management) to stop transmission from human to human. All four suspected cases of infection were isolated immediately after being suspected of having SARS. All close contacts were quarantined. This control strategy seems to be working: there were no cases acquired in the community between 30 January 2004 and the summer of 2004 when this text went to press. Although it would be premature to confirm that a SARS outbreak was circumvented due to the strict control of the wildlife markets, the drastic measures of the local authorities were indispensable with regard to prevention of an emergent infectious disease. Whether the control of wildlife market was the key to avoiding the source of SARS transmission requires further verification.

5.4 Two laboratory acquired cases

With regards to the second SARS event, a young postgraduate working at an institute of virology in Beijing from 7 to 22 March 2004, developed symptoms of pneumonia on 25 March. When she returned home to Hefei, the capital city of Anhui Province, she was diagnosed as having SARS and transmitted the disease to 7 others including her parents and healthcare workers both in Beijing and Hefei. Twenty-three days later, another person working at the same institute presented with the same symptoms, also diagnosed as SARS. It has been confirmed that these two separate cases arose from the same contaminated laboratory and did not infect each other (incubation period 2–10 days). The institute was shut down immediately. In addition to the isolation of 9 SARS cases, more than 200 contacts were quarantined. Fortunately, there was no further outbreak from this event of SARS (Fig. 5.2).

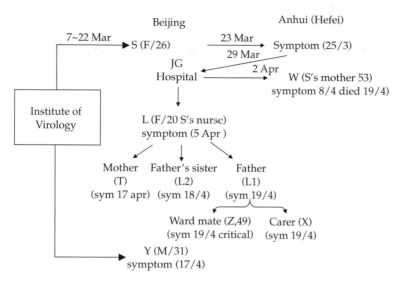

Figure 5.2 The second event of SARS between March and April 2004.

Laboratory acquired cases in other countries are described in Chapter 15 in this volume.

5.5 Conclusions

SARS has not been eradicated and humans remain vulnerable. To-date, SARS vaccines and SARS-specific therapy are still under research. The most effective way for prophylaxis is cutting off the transmission route and blocking the epidemic from breaking out. Three major aspects stay extraordinarily instructive: the Four-earliness policy, strict control of wildlife markets, and strict laboratory bio-safety regulations.

CHAPTER 6

Confronting SARS: a view from Hong Kong

J. S. Malik Peiris and Yi Guan

6.1 Summary

Severe acute respiratory syndrome (SARS) emerged as a new disease in Guangdong province, People's Republic of China in late 2002. Within weeks it had spread to Hong Kong and thence globally to affect over 25 countries across five continents. The disease had the propensity to cause clusters of pneumonia particularly in healthcare workers or close family contacts. A global effort coordinated by the World Health Organization (WHO) successfully defined the aetiology, epidemiology, and clinical characteristics of the disease and the implementation of case identification, isolation, and infection control measures led to the interruption of the global outbreak by July 2003. The pattern of disease emergence and strategies for control of SARS provide lessons for coping with future emerging infectious disease threats.

6.2 Emergence of a new disease

News of an outbreak of 'atypical pneumonia' circulating in Guangdong province reached Hong Kong in early February 2003. Residents in Guangzhou, the provincial capital of Guangdong, were reportedly rushing to buy masks, antibiotics, and traditional remedies including white vinegar, the boiling of which was believed to ward of respiratory infections (Rosling and Rosling 2003). At this time, the health authorities of the Hong Kong Special Administrative Region (SAR) and Guangdong did not have efficient channels for exchanging information on matters of health on a 'real-time' basis (SARS Expert Committee 2003).

By 11 February, the People's Republic of China had informed the WHO of an outbreak of an acute respiratory syndrome with 305 cases and 5 deaths in Guangdong province (WHO 2003c). The disease had been circulating in Guangdong since November 2002. It was a severe viral pneumonia, that failed to respond to antibiotics including beta-lactams and macrolides. The most notable characteristic was the propensity to cause clusters of disease in family contacts and healthcare workers and in recognition of this, the disease had been named 'infectious atypical pneumonia' (Zhong and Zeng 2003). Some of the patients with this disease in Guangdong during November and December 2002 had a history of occupational or other exposure to markets or restaurants involved in the live game animal trade (Breiman et al. 2003; Zhong et al. 2003). A number of aetiological agents were under consideration including chlamydia.

6.3 Surveillance and aetiology

In response to this information, on 14 February the Hospital Authority and Department of Health in Hong Kong set up surveillance for cases of severe atypical pneumonia admitted to public hospitals. The Hospital Authority of Hong Kong manages all public hospitals accounting for >90% of all hospital admissions within Hong Kong SAR. However, community acquired pneumonia is a common disease in all parts of the world and Hong Kong SAR (population 6.8 million) had around 1400 episodes of disease every month, with 55–75 of them requiring management in intensive care units (SARS Expert Committee 2003). It was clear from the outset that an indicator with such a high baseline would not provide early warning of a new disease. Therefore, surveillance focussed on severe community acquired pneumonia and included intensive microbiological investigation of all such cases. Those patients with recent travel to Guangdong received particular attention, though microbiological investigation was not restricted to this group.

By mid-February, aetiological diagnoses in patients with atypical pneumonia in Hong Kong included *Chlamydia psittaci, Chlamydia pneumoniae,* adenovirus, parainfluenza, rickettsia, influenza A, influenza B, mycoplasma, and pyogenic bacterial infections. However, there was nothing remarkable in these findings that would explain the unusual outbreak of disease in adjoining Guangdong. Furthermore, there was no significant difference in pattern of aetiological agents in patients with or without a history of recent travel to Mainland China. The first finding of note came on 20 February with influenza A subtype H5N1 being isolated from two members of the same family who had returned to Hong Kong from a visit to Fujian (WHO 2003c; Peiris *et al.* 2004). After the 'bird flu' outbreak in 1997, this was the first time that H5N1 viruses had been isolated from humans. In the context of the ongoing pneumonic disease of unknown aetiology in Guangdong, the WHO and its influenza network activated emergency pandemic response plans.

However, intensive investigation of other patients in Hong Kong, as well as some clinical specimens from patients in Guangzhou investigated in collaboration with Prof Zhong Nan San (Zhong *et al.* 2003) revealed no further cases of influenza A (H5N1) infection. Some patients had evidence of influenza A (H3N2) infection. The possibility of a reassortant human H3N2 virus that had acquired the internal genes of an avian virus or the emergence of a drift mutant was considered. Genetic analysis of these isolates from Guangdong did not reveal such reassortment.

On 26 February, there were reports of an outbreak of respiratory disease in healthcare workers in a hospital in Hanoi. Carlo Urbani, the WHO epidemiologist who alerted WHO to that cluster of cases, sadly succumbed to the disease himself. By 11 March, a large cluster of cases was being reported from the Prince of Wales Hospital in Hong Kong (Lee *et al.* 2003). Within Hong Kong, our own efforts focussed on patients with pneumonia outside of that large cluster of cases at Prince of Wales Hospital. In response to these outbreaks, WHO issued a global alert on 12 March (WHO 2003c). By 14 March, further clusters of patients were reported in Singapore and Toronto. By 15 March, WHO had received over 150 reports of this new disease from outside of Mainland China. The disease was named (SARS), a preliminary case definition was provided and WHO issued a travel advisory warning against travel to affected regions.

On 17 March, WHO initiated a network of laboratories across the world to help establish the aetiology of this new disease. The network functioned through daily teleconferences exchanging information on patients and specimens being investigated on a real-time basis. In addition, a secure website was established to post findings that could be shared by members within the network (WHO 2003d). The overall clinical picture and the lack of a response to antibiotics suggested a viral cause. The clinical features of the disease have been described in detail elsewhere and will not be reviewed here (Lee *et al.* 2003; Peiris *et al.* 2003; Tsang *et al.* 2003; Jerigan *et al.* 2004). Conventional microbiologic investigations failed to reveal an aetiological explanation for the illness in these patients with suspected SARS. Similar findings were being echoed by members of the WHO network laboratories who were investigating patients from Vietnam, Singapore, Toronto, and Germany. As a result, we turned our search to look for novel viral pathogens.

By 18 March, laboratories within the WHO laboratory network reported sighting of Paramyxovirus-like particles by direct electron microscopy on respiratory specimens from patients with SARS. In addition, detection of human metapneumovirus RNA in clinical specimens by Reverse transcription-Polymerase chain reaction (RT-PCR) were reported from laboratories in Hong Kong and Toronto. Between 21 and 24 March, three laboratories within the WHO network of laboratories including our own, independently reported the isolation of a novel coronavirus associated with SARS (Drosten *et al.* 2003; Ksiazek *et al.* 2003; Peiris *et al.* 2003*a*).

In our own laboratory, the strategy in searching for a novel virus associated with SARS included the use of consensus primer or low stringency based RT-PCR to search for viruses related to, though not identical with known viral pathogen groups, random RT-PCR methods, the use of cell lines not usually used for diagnosing conventional respiratory viruses, and electron microscopy on tissue specimens, when available. One of the cell-lines included in our panel of cells was FRhK-4—a cell used to grow hepatitis A virus. Over the past year, we had found FRhK-4 cells able to support the replication of a number of respiratory viruses including human metapneumovirus, a virus with fastidious growth requirements (Peiris *et al.* 2003*c*). A lung biopsy from one patient and a nasopharyngeal aspirate from another showed evidence of a subtle cytopathic effect on FRhK-4 cells which became more pronounced on passage (Fig. 6.1(a)). Using infected cells as antigen in an indirect immunoflourescence assay (Fig. 6.1(b)), we were able to demonstrate seroconversion or rising antibody titres in sera of a number of patients with suspected SARS. Paired sera from patients with atypical pneumonia due to other causes were seronegative. Thus there was a close link between the novel virus and SARS. Thin section

electron microscopy on infected cells clearly showed evidence of abundant virus particles in the golgi-ER complex and on the surface of infected cells. Electron microscopy of infected cell supernatants using negative staining showed evidence of virus particles of 60–80 nm with a morphology compatible with coronaviruses. Electron microscopic examination of the lung biopsy that yielded the virus isolate revealed viral particles similar in morphology to that seen in virus infected cells *in vitro*. Genetic sequencing of gene products amplified by random RT-PCR differentially expressed on infected and un-infected cells yielded a 624 bp fragment of genetic sequence with homology to the replicase gene of the Coronaviridae. However, the extent of genetic homology to known coronaviruses was not high and we suspected that we were dealing with a novel coronavirus (Peiris *et al.* 2003*a*). We established evidence of SARS-CoV infection by serology or RT-PCR in 45 of 50 patients with SARS whereas there was little evidence of virus activity in community controls (Peiris *et al.* 2003*a*). These findings provided evidence of the association between this novel coronavirus and SARS. Using Vero-E6 cells, similar findings were being reported to the WHO laboratory network from the Centers for Disease Control, Atlanta and the Bernhard Nocht Institute for Tropical Medicine, Hamburg who were investigating patients originating from Vietnam and Singapore, respectively (Drosten *et al.* 2003; Ksiazek *et al.* 2003).

(a) 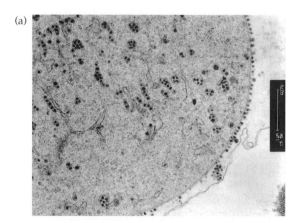   (b)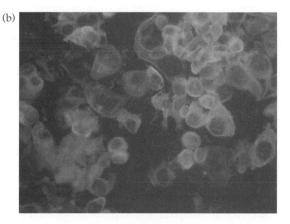

Figure 6.1 (a) Thin section electron micrograph of FRhK-4 cells infected with SARS coronavirus (acknowledgements to J. M. Nicholls). (b) Shows convalescent serum from a patient with SARS reacting in an indirect immunofluorescence test with SARS-coronavirus-infected FRhK-4 cells.

Independent reports of a novel coronavirus from three laboratories investigating patients from three countries provided a compelling case for the link between the novel virus, now named SARS coronavirus (SARS-CoV) and SARS. Confirmation of Koch's postulates was achieved by reproducing the disease in cynomolgous macaques following experimental inoculation with SARS-CoV (Fouchier *et al.* 2003; Kuiken *et al.* 2003a; reviewed by Osterhaus in Chapter 7, this volume). The full genetic sequence of the SARS-CoV was unravelled within weeks of its initial isolation providing the biological foundation for further research on antivirals, vaccines, and pathogenesis (Marra *et al.* 2003; Rota *et al.* 2003).

6.4 Laboratory diagnosis

The identification of the SARS-CoV as the presumptive aetiological agent of SARS immediately provided two options for laboratory diagnosis—a serological test, initially based on indirect immunofluorescence on virus-infected cells, and an RT-PCR test based on the partial genetic sequence then available. Initial indirect immunofluorescent tests with blood donor sera on SARS-CoV infected cells gave negative results suggesting that SARS-CoV was not previously endemic in the human population (Ksiazek *et al.* 2003; Peiris *et al.* 2003a). It also indicated that the immunofluorescent test could be a useful serological test for diagnosis of SARS. On 28 March, just a week after the aetiological agent was identified, we commenced providing a laboratory testing for SARS based on these two tests with the caveat that these were experimental tests still under evaluation. Under normal circumstances, one would not provide a diagnostic service without careful prior evaluation and validation. However, these times were far from 'normal'—the need for the diagnostic service was here and now, not sometime in the future, when the test may be better validated but the need may have passed. But providing such a diagnostic service was fraught with problems. We were swamped with diagnostic test requests from across Hong Kong with over 200 specimens arriving per day at our laboratory alone. There were initially two and then three laboratories providing serology

and RT-PCR diagnosis. Clinical data on many of these patients were difficult to obtain and therefore evaluation of the performance characteristics of the tests on a real-time basis proved difficult. In general, data-capture and data-flow proved to be a major obstacle in reacting to the SARS crisis. The sudden and large workload hampered further optimization and test development in the short-term. In subsequent months, the Hospital Authority of Hong Kong had consolidated all the clinical and laboratory data into one database (designated e-SARS) thereby facilitating much better data analysis. Such a system would be invaluable in dealing with emerging infectious disease outbreaks in future.

It became clear that while serology was reliable at providing retrospective diagnosis of SARS within the context of this outbreak, diagnosis early in the illness was difficult to achieve. Seroconversion only occurred around day 10 of disease or later. Surprisingly, RT-PCR for SARS-CoV yielded more positive results later in the course of the illness when compared with the first 5 days of illness (Poon *et al.* 2003a,b). This contrasts with other respiratory viral infections where viral detection rates decrease in later stages of disease. Thus, these first generation SARS-CoV tests had limited value in screening patients suspected with SARS for purposes of triage.

6.5 Epidemiology and control

Within weeks of SARS appearing in Hong Kong, a travel and business hub for the region, the disease had spread to affect over 8000 patients in 26 countries across 5 continents. Hospitals served as amplifiers of the disease and SARS exposed the logistical problems of coping with an epidemic of infectious disease in the twenty-first century and highlighted the weak links in infection control within hospitals, especially in tertiary hospitals providing modern intensive care. Determined and concerted global public health measures by case detection using a clinical case definition and patient isolation, succeeded in interrupting the chain of disease transmission and by 5 July 2003, the outbreak was formally declared as over. The understanding of the aetiology and the availability of diagnostic tests no doubt contributed to this success. But it is not clear whether the public health interventions may have achieved the desired result irrespective of such knowledge and activity. However, a better understanding of the causative virus did prove invaluable in a number of respects that were pertinent for control of SARS. Virus was isolated from the faeces and urine as well as the respiratory tract suggesting that the infection was not confined to the respiratory tract. Furthermore, since SARS-CoV was unusually stable in the environment including faeces (WHO 2003*m*), the possibility of faecal transmission had to be considered. These findings provided the basis for understanding the community outbreak at Amoy gardens where over 300 patients were infected within a few days and where contaminated sewage may have played a role in transmission of infection (Department of Health, Hong Kong SAR 2003). Quantitative RT-PCR assays on longitudinally collected specimens from the same patient showed that SARS-CoV viral load in the upper respiratory tract was low in the first 5 days of illness and increased progressively to peak at around day 10 after disease onset (Peiris *et al.* 2003*e*). This was in contrast to most other respiratory viral infections where maximal viral load in the respiratory tract occurs soon after the onset of clinical disease. These findings explained the epidemiological observations that transmission was more common after the first 5 days of illness (Lipsitch *et al.* 2003). The unusual stability of SARS-CoV may also explain the propensity of this virus to spread so readily in a hospital setting. The low viral load in respiratory secretions early in the disease suggested that diagnostic tests applied to upper respiratory tract specimens would have to be pushed to the limits of sensitivity in order to diagnose disease in the first few days when viral loads are very low. Later modifications of RT-PCR test strategies based on real-time RT-PCR together with enhanced RNA extraction methods allowed higher success rates in diagnosis of patients in the first few days of illness (Poon *et al.* 2003*b*).

6.6 Animal origins

The fact that there was little serological evidence of SARS-CoV in the general population indicated that this was a virus of animal origin that transmitted to humans relatively recently. The anecdotal reports of the early patients with SARS having contact with the live wild animal restaurant trade suggested that live wild game markets that were prevalent in Guangdong and other parts of Mainland China may be the initial source of the virus infecting humans. Investigation of these wild game markets revealed the presence of a closely related virus in a number of small mammalian species, most notably, the palm civet cat. Persons working directly in this trade had high prevalence of antibody to the SARS-CoV and related animal viruses (Guan *et al.* 2003). The re-emergence of SARS in humans in early 2004 was also linked to the animal trade (described in Chapter 5, this volume).

6.7 What next? Lessons from SARS

It is interesting that the techniques that played the key roles in identification of the aetiological agent of SARS in all three laboratories were the traditional methods of cell culture and electron microscopy (Drosten *et al.* 2003; Ksiazek *et al.* 2003; Peiris *et al.* 2003*a*). Similar strategies were instrumental in the discovery of other recent novel pathogens including Nipah virus and human metapneumovirus. In this age of high throughput genomics, it is important that expertise in methods of 'classical virology' are not neglected and lost. Given budgetary constraints imposed by 'managed care' and repeated 'efficiency gains' in the health systems of many countries, there is the perceived need for diagnostic virology laboratories to be primarily accountable for patient care (i.e. providing rapid diagnosis) rather than for public health. Therefore, conventional technologies such as viral culture are being abandoned in favour of methods that provide rapid diagnosis such as antigen detection and molecular (e.g. RT-PCR based) diagnosis. The latter methods only detect the presence of a pre-selected agent—they are not 'open ended' methods able to detect the unexpected! It is, however, equally clear that once the candidate agent had been identified, the approaches of modern molecular biology made short shrift of the complete genetic characterization of the virus.

In the context of increasing pre-occupation with bio-terrorist threats, SARS reminds us that 'Nature' remains the greatest bio-terrorist threat of all. It is desirable that the funds and resources pouring into combating bio-terrorism be targeted generically, in ways that help our capacity to confront the certainty of naturally emerging infectious diseases as well as uncertain possibilities of bio-terrorist attacks. Most recent emerging infectious disease threats have been zoonoses arising from microbe crossing species barrier to humans (Osterhaus 2001).

SARS vividly illustrated that we indeed live in a global village in relation to emerging infectious disease. SARS also illustrated that emerging infectious diseases are not just threats to human health but can radically impact on the economy and society as a whole. Given the rapid dissemination of SARS through air-travel (described and modelled in chapter 11, this volume.), its control required a coordinated and global response. WHO was able to mobilize and coordinate a rapid global response that was instrumental in understanding and controlling SARS. The speed and extent of success of such intervention is dependent on national governments.

SARS manifested a number of features that made it more amenable to control through public health measures than some other potential emerging infectious disease threats. Most important of these was the fact that there was little or no transmission of SARS-CoV in the late incubation period or even in the first few days of illness. Furthermore, asymptomatic infection seemed to be less common and less epidemiologically relevant than with many other respiratory viral infections. It is salutary to keep in mind that the next global emerging infectious disease threat may not be so amenable to interruption by case detection and isolation, once human to human transmission is established. The current threat from avian influenza subtype H5N1, is a case in point (WHO 2004a). The parallels with SARS are poignant. As with SARS in late 2002, there are now repeated interspecies transmission events of H5N1 virus from the avian reservoir to humans and other mammalian species. In this instance, the intensity and geographical scale over which these events are occurring are vastly greater than was the case with SARS. 'Wet markets' where live animals are sold for human consumption play a role in both diseases (Guan *et al.* 2003; Webster 2004). At the time of writing, transmission of influenza H5N1 to humans is inefficient, and has so far, not resulted in efficient human to human transmission. However, if left unchecked, as occurred with SARS in late 2002, it is possible that the virus may acquire the property of efficient human–human transmission, either through reassortment or mutation of the viral genome. Once adapted to human–human transmission, influenza is highly transmissible, both in the late incubation period as well as early in the disease. Therefore, its spread may not be amenable to interruption with the same public health measures used to successfully contain SARS. The recent reports that the influenza pandemic of 1918 may have been caused by an avian virus directly adapting to human transmission (rather than reassorting with a pre-existing human virus) provides an ominous portent (Stevens 2004).

Acknowledgements

This chapter is dedicated to the healthcare professionals in Hong Kong and elsewhere who risked their lives in the service of their profession, some of them making the ultimate sacrifice.

Our own colleagues who played a key role in the discovery of the aetiology of SARS, in developing diagnostic tests and in unravelling some of its mysteries include K. H. Chan, J. M. Nicholls, L. L. M. Poon, W. L. Lim, V. C. C. Cheng, C. M. Chu, K. S. Chan, I. F. Hung, S. T. Lai, T. K. Ng, W. H. Seto, D. Tsang, L. Yam, B. J. Zheng, R. Yung, K. Y. Yuen, and many others in The University of Hong Kong, the Hospital Authority of Hong Kong, and the Department of Health, Hong Kong SAR.

CHAPTER 7

The aetiology of SARS: Koch's postulates fulfilled

Albert D. M. E. Osterhaus, Ron A. M. Fouchier, and Thijs Kuiken

7.1 Summary

Proof that a newly identified coronavirus, severe acute respiratory syndrome coronavirus (SARS-CoV) is the primary cause of severe acute respiratory syndrome (SARS) came from a series of studies on experimentally infected cynomolgus macaques (*Macaca fascicularis*). SARS-CoV-infected macaques developed a disease comparable to SARS in humans; the virus was re-isolated from these animals and they developed SARS-CoV-specific antibodies. This completed the fulfilment of Koch's postulates, as modified by Rivers for viral diseases, for SARS-CoV as the aetiological agent of SARS. Besides the macaque model, a ferret and a cat model for SARS-CoV were also developed. These animal models allow comparative pathogenesis studies for SARS-CoV infections and testing of different intervention strategies. The first of these studies has shown that pegylated interferon-α, a drug approved for human use, limits SARS-CoV replication and lung damage in experimentally infected macaques. Finally, we argue that, given the worldwide nature of the socio-economic changes that have predisposed for the emergence of SARS and avian influenza in Southeast Asia, such changes herald the beginning of a global trend for which we are ill prepared.

7.2 Identifying the causative agent of SARS

SARS emerged in late 2002 as a new human disease entity (Lee *et al.* 2003; WHO 2003*e*), resulting in more than 800 deaths from more than 8000 documented probable cases of the disease. About 6 months after the disease was first recognized, the World Health Organization (WHO) declared this global outbreak to be under control, with only a few sporadic cases having been diagnosed since. In response to the start of the outbreak, the WHO coordinated an international collaboration that included clinical, epidemiological, and laboratory investigations to control the expanding epidemic. Identification of the causative agents was one of the first research priorities. Several viruses and bacteria were initially identified in SARS patients. The recently identified human metapneumovirus (hMPV) (van den Hoogen *et al.* 2001) and a newly discovered human coronavirus, SARS-CoV (Drosten *et al.* 2003) proved to be the most likely candidates on epidemiological grounds in a comparative study involving more than 300 patients fitting the WHO SARS case definition in 12 cohorts in Asia and Europe. hMPV infection was diagnosed in 12% and SARS-CoV infection in 75% of the patients. Other respiratory pathogens were identified only sporadically. SARS-CoV was therefore the most likely causal agent of SARS (Kuiken *et al.* 2003*a*). According to Koch's postulates, as modified by Rivers (1937) for virus diseases, six criteria should be met to establish a virus as the cause of a disease. The first three of these, namely isolation of the virus from diseased hosts, cultivation in host cells, and proof of filterability, were met for both by hMPV and SARS-CoV. The remaining three criteria were tested for in a series of experiments that we conducted in cynomolgus macaques (*M. fascicularis*): production of a comparable disease in the original host species or a related one, re-isolation of the virus, and detection of a specific immunoresponse to the virus (Kuiken *et al.* 2003*a*). Four monkeys were infected with a SARS-CoV isolated in Vero cells from a patient who had died of SARS in Hong Kong. Three of these became lethargic from days 2 to 3 onwards after infection and two of them developed a temporary skin rash at day 4 after infection. Upon necropsy, carried out on day 6 after infection, three of the animals had multiple foci of pulmonary consolidation in both lungs. Histologically, the main lesions in the consolidated lung tissue involved the alveoli and bronchioles, and consisted of areas with acute or more advanced phases of diffused alveolar damage. Occasional multinucleated giant cells were found. In the macaque without clear macroscopic pulmonary lesions, minimum multifocal inflammatory lesions were observed histologically in the pulmonary tissue. By immunohistochemistry, the presence of SARS-CoV could be demonstrated in inflamed lung tissue of the three macaques showing pulmonary consolidation. The presence of SARS-CoV in the lungs was also confirmed by showing typical coronavirus-like particles in pneumocytes in affected pulmonary areas. From day 2 onwards after infection, SARS-CoV could be isolated or demonstrated by reverse transcription–polymerase chain reaction (RT-PCR) in sputum, nasal swabs, and pharyngeal swabs of one or more animals. In a separate macaque infection experiment, it was shown that SARS-CoV-neutralizing antibodies were present from day 12 onwards after infection (Fouchier *et al.* 2003). The virus was also isolated from the faeces of one of the two monkeys involved in this experiment. No other relevant respiratory pathogens were identified in any of the macaques experimentally infected with SARS-CoV. Collectively, these data completed the six criteria that needed to be fulfilled to identify SARS-CoV as the aetiological agent of SARS, which probably spilled over recently from an animal reservoir. Moreover, lesions in macaques infected experimentally with hMPV, isolated from a non-SARS individual, were limited to mild suppurative rhinitis and minimal erosions in conducting airways (Kuiken *et al.* 2003*a*, 2004). The disease was not exacerbated in two SARS-CoV-infected macaques that were subsequently inoculated with hMPV (Fouchier *et al.* 2003; Kuiken *et al.* 2003*a*). Besides cynomolgus macaques, we also succeeded in infecting ferrets and domestic cats experimentally with SARS-CoV (Martina *et al.* 2003). The virus was efficiently transmitted to non-infected cage mates. The cats did not develop clinical signs, whereas some of the ferrets became lethargic and one died. Infection of the respiratory tract was evident in all the infected animals and, histologically, SARS-CoV infection was associated with pulmonary lesions similar to those observed in the SARS-CoV-infected macaques, except that they were milder, particularly in the cats. The availability of three animal models for SARS-CoV infection now allows us to carry out comparative pathogenesis studies as well as the testing of different intervention strategies like the use of antivirals, SARS-CoV-specific antibodies, and candidate vaccines. Currently, we are using the ferret and the macaque models for such studies. Recently, we showed in the macaque model that prophylactic treatment of SARS-CoV-infected macaques with the antiviral agent pegylated interferon-α, a drug approved for human use, significantly reduces viral replication and excretion as well as pulmonary damage, compared with untreated macaques (Haagmans *et al.* 2004). Post-exposure treatment with this drug yielded intermediate results. These data warrant clinical studies with this drug, if and when SARS re-emerges. Prophylactic or early post-exposure treatment with pegylated interferon-α may help reduce the impact of SARS-CoV infections on healthcare workers and others possibly exposed to SARS-CoV, and may limit the spread of the virus in the human population. Finally, one may wonder whether the recent emergence of SARS and the emergence of avian influenza A outbreaks, which also have resulted in animal to human transmissions with fatal consequences (de Jong *et al.* 1997; Claas and Osterhaus 1998; Webby and Webster 2004; Hien *et al.* 2004), in Southeast Asia and more particularly in Guandong Province of China, may be a result of key socio-economic changes in that region (T. Kuiken and A. D. M. E. Osterhaus, unpublished data). It may be argued that given the worldwide nature of these changes, the observed increase in the emergence of such virus infections in this area may herald the beginning of a global trend for which we are ill prepared (Kuiken *et al.* 2003*b*, 2004).

CHAPTER 8

Laboratory diagnosis of SARS

Alison Bermingham, Paul P. Heinen, Miren Hurriza-Gómara, Jim J. Gray, Hazel Appleton, and Maria C. Zambon

8.1 Summary

The emergence of new viral infections of man requires the development of robust diagnostic tests that can be applied in the differential diagnosis of acute illness, or to determine past exposure so as to establish the true burden of the disease. Since the recognition in April 2003 of the severe acute respiratory syndrome coronavirus (SARS-CoV) as the causative agent of the syndrome of SARS, enormous efforts have been applied to develop molecular and serological tests for SARS which can assist rapid detection of cases, accurate diagnosis of illness, and the application of control measures. International progress in the laboratory diagnosis of SARS-CoV infection during acute illness has led to internationally agreed WHO (World Health Organization) criteria for the confirmation of SARS. Developments in the dissection of the human immune response to SARS indicates that serological tests on convalescent sera are essential to confirm SARS infection given the sub-optimal predictive value of molecular detection tests carried out during acute SARS illness.

8.2 Introduction

Recognition of the newly described SARS-CoV followed from its detection in clinical material from humans affected with SARS in 2003 (Drosten et al. 2003; Peiris et al. 2003a; Rota et al. 2003). The identification of the virus and its relationship to human disease were confirmed using Koch's postulates modified for viral diseases and was achieved through an international network of laboratories working under the coordination of the WHO (Kuiken et al. 2003a). Experimental work has indicated that the SARS-CoV can be recovered from several organs in infected animals, indicating a disseminated infection, which parallels the observational experience of many of the laboratories involved in handling clinical samples from SARS cases (Peiris et al. 2003b). The main site of replication, pathology, and recovery of the virus during human infection is considered to be the lower respiratory tract (Nicholls et al. 2003). This is consistent with the most important route of human to human transmission being through respiratory secretions, although outbreaks of infection which involved dissemination of virus excreted in faeces have also been described (Peiris et al. 2003b). Accurate laboratory diagnosis of SARS-CoV is essential to ensure appropriate individual patient management, local infection control, and public health measures which were critical in halting the global spread of the first serious new threat to the human population in the twenty-first century.

One of the difficulties of accurate clinical diagnosis of SARS is the relatively long incubation period following infection (mean 6–7 days) but ranging up to 10–14 days, prior to the onset of clinical symptoms and the relatively non-specific nature of the initial illness presentation. Early symptoms include fever, chills, non-specific malaise, and myalgia compared with more florid respiratory symptoms which develop later during illness associated with pulmonary infiltrates in the lungs (Donnelly et al. 2003). Summary analyses of published cases series indicate that between 25% and 75% of cases demonstrate gastrointestinal symptoms of diaorrhoea, nausea, and vomiting as illness progresses (Jernigan *et al.* 2004) The wide range of recognized gastrointestinal disturbance in different case series may be a reflection of the fact that the earliest compilations of data of the disease did not fully recognize this clinical feature. Overall, the major clinical symptoms of respiratory and enteric disease caused by the SARS-CoV in humans are analogous to disease syndromes caused by several animal coronaviruses in their natural hosts.

8.3 Clinical virology

Clinical studies on SARS have shed light on the diagnostic usefulness of different samples at different times during illness, summarized in Fig. 8.1. In many viral illnesses, virus shedding is greatest during the early symptomatic phase of illness, around the onset of symptoms, for example, influenza (Hayden *et al.* 1998). However, in the case of SARS-CoV, virus excretion is comparatively low during the initial phase of illness and it is necessary to use very sensitive tests that are able to detect low levels of viral nucleic acid during the first days of illness. The mainstay of diagnosis during the illness phase of SARS has involved the use of reverse transcription-polymyrase chain reaction (RT-PCR) to detect the SARS-CoV nucleic acid amplified directly from clinical samples. RT-PCR protocols were developed with unprecedented speed as a result of the efforts of the WHO collaborative laboratory network. Samples of different body fluids such as blood, respiratory secretions, urine, stool, and lung tissue from suspected and probable cases of SARS were analysed. The end point of detection for the SARS-CoV was similar to that found in previously described protocols for detection of known human CoVs (Vabret *et al.* 2001).

It is clear that viral load increases in respiratory samples in the second week of SARS illness (Peiris *et al.* 2003b), and that the viral load is greatest in samples taken from the lower respiratory tract (Drosten *et al.* 2003), peaking around day 10, with the peak of viral detection in faeces coming slightly later. SARS-CoV RNA was detected in only 32% of individuals in nasopharyngeal aspirates at initial presentation (mean 3.2 days after illness onset) but in 68% at day 14 (Peiris *et al.* 2003b), and in over 90% of faecal samples collected in the second week of illness, peaking around days 15–17 (Chan *et al.* 2004). Quantification indicated that viral load in respiratory secretions peaked at day 10 with a geometric mean titre of 1.9×10^7 copies per ml. The clinical features of SARS illness therefore appear to be a good reflection of the body compartments/fluids in which SARS virus has been detected or recovered, with a clear time course. The detection of virus replication in different body compartments over several weeks,

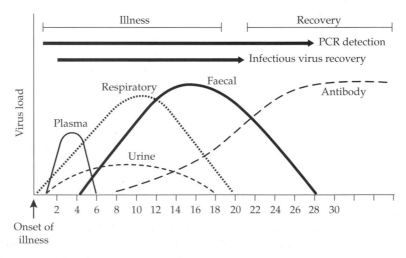

Figure 8.1 Schematic diagram of the course of virus shedding and detection in body fluids during SARS illness and recovery. Onset of illness is taken to be the onset of symptomatic fever.

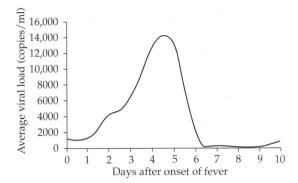

Figure 8.2 Schematic diagram of the detection of SARS viral RNA using RT-PCR in plasma in early SARS illness. Compiled from Grant *et al.* (2003).

prior to resolution or progression to death, underlies the suggested use of different clinical samples to detect virus at different time points after illness onset (Fig. 8.1). More recently, analysis of sequential samples of plasma from SARS patients early during illness using PCR indicates that there is an early peak of viraemia, with up to 70% of samples containing detectable virus in the first few days post onset of illness (Fig. 8.2; Grant *et al.* 2003). This suggests that a viraemic phase is then most likely followed by increasing virus replication in the lower airways and gastrointestinal tract. Taken together, these observations indicate that sampling to detect SARS-CoV in the first week post onset of illness should involve the simultaneous collection and analysis of different clinical samples including respiratory samples from as low in the respiratory tract as is practicable, blood, faeces, and urine. Detection of virus in the second week after the onset of illness is actually more likely, given the higher viral load, and should also involve sampling from multiple sites.

8.4 Molecular detection

Despite reasonably high rates of detection of virus in clinical samples, and good analytical sensitivity of the tests themselves, the predictive value of molecular diagnostic tests in the early stages of illness are still sub-optimal as they cannot rule out the presence of SARS-CoV. This is partly a reflection of the variable viral load in clinical samples,

particularly in respiratory samples which are most likely to be taken from the upper respiratory tract where the priority is to minimize aerosol generation when sampling in order to prevent infection of health care workers. This and the fact that viral replication does not appear to peak until some time after the onset of disease may result in sub-optimal samples. Obtaining a clear diagnosis may be difficult when the disease symptoms are least specific.

Parallel testing of samples for other infectious agents such as influenza, Mycoplasma pneumoniae, Legionella pneumophila, and human metapneumovirus, which are capable of causing a similar clinical syndrome is essential in the differential diagnosis early after disease onset and may help to exclude SARS, particularly in returning travellers from countries where SARS is considered likely to re-emerge from an animal reservoir, although co-infection of SARS with other respiratory pathogens can occur (Poutanen *et al.* 2003). If the presence of an alternative diagnosis is to be used as the justification for discontinuing SARS-specific isolation procedures, the diagnosis should be based on tests with a high predictive value and the clinical illness should be fully explainable by the alternative diagnosis. Testing of multiple sequential samples increases the reliability of laboratory diagnosis, and reduces the likelihood of false-positive results, which is always of concern when using sensitive molecular diagnostic techniques. These findings underlie the current stringent WHO recommendations regarding the confirmation and quality control of SARS laboratory diagnosis, 'Laboratories performing SARS specific PCR tests should adopt strict criteria for confirmation of positive results, especially in low prevalence areas where the predictive values might be lower' (Galen and Gambino 1975). This guidance includes the current requirement for detection of virus by RT-PCR in two different samples (e.g. respiratory and faecal), or sequential samples from the same body site on different days and robust confirmatory strategies. Examples of laboratory acquired infection which occurred in Southeast Asia in 2003/2004, leading to extensive deployment of health care resources for contact tracing and quarantine, emphasize the necessity of stringent bio-safety considerations in laboratories conducting SARS diagnosis.

8.5 Virus targets for diagnosis

Initial diagnostic work focussed on the molecular detection of SARS-CoV *RdRp* (*Pol*) gene, because the *Pol* gene sequences were the first available (Drosten, *et al.* 2003), and the *Pol* region of the coronavirus genome is well conserved across all coronaviruses. The use of detection probes involving degenerate primer sets which can detect all known coronaviruses (Stephensen *et al.* 1999) remains a useful screening approach, because this allows the deployment of a pan-corona molecular strategy, which will detect all known human coronaviruses, some of which may possibly cause diseases that overlap with the clinical syndrome of SARS. This approach can be run in parallel with RT-PCRs that are absolutely specific for SARS-CoV (Yam *et al.* 2003). The sequence conservation in the

Pol region across all coronaviruses is such that diagnostic SARS-CoV tests based on the *Pol* region of the genome should, as part of a validation process, exclude detection of 229E (Group 1 coronaviruses) and OC43 (Group 2 coronaviruses) to avoid false positive detections of human coronaviruses.

Coronaviruses have unusually long RNA genomes of ca. 30,000 bases. Viral replication and transcription is complex. As data have developed about the nature of SARS-CoV replication in vitro, it is evident that there is a transcription gradient across the viral genome, in common with other coronaviruses (Thiel *et al.* 2003). The genomic organization of the coronavirus, with the non-structural genes at the 5′-end and structural genes at the 3′-end, reflects this transcription strategy. Differential transcription generates a gradient of

Table 8.1 Detection of SARS-CoV in spiked simulated clinical specimens using different molecular detection strategies

Sample type	Number of samples	*Pol* Degenerate Primers 2Bp/4Bm[1] (Block)	N5/N6 Primers[2] (Block)	N5/N6 Primers[3] (Light cycler)	N Primers[4] (Light cycler)	SARS specific Pol Primers[5] (Light cycler)
SARS-CoV spiked samples(%)						
Faecal[a]	38	15 (39.5%)	28 (73.7%)	32 (84.2 %)	32 (84.2%)	30 (78.9%)
Plasma	15	13 (86.7%)	14 (93.3%)	15 (100%)	15 (100%)	15 (100%)
Respiratory[b]	35	34 (97.1%)	27 (77.1%)	28 (80.0%)	30 (85.7%)	28 (80%)
Urine	9	7 (77.8%)	8 (88.9%)	9 (100%)	9 (100%)	9 (100%)
Total spiked	97	69 (71.1%)	77 (79.4%)	84 (86.6%)	86 (88.7%)	82 (84.5%)
Negative controls						
Negative faecal	12	12	0	0	1	2
Negative plasma	5	0	0	0	0	0
Negative respiratory	5	5	0	0	1	2
Negative urine	1	0	0	0	0	0
Total negative	23	17	0	0	2	4
Overall sensitivity (%)		71.1%	79.4%	86.6%	88.7%	84.5%
Overall specificity (%)		57.5%	100%	100%	92%	85.2%
Positive predictive Value		80.2%	100%	100%	97.7%	95.3%

[a] 12 out of 38 faecal samples were co-inoculated with rotavirus

[b] 14 out of 35 respiratory samples were co-inoculated with influenza A virus

Notes:

[1] Stephensen *et al.* 1999.

[2] SARS specific nucleocapsid primers N5 - 5′ GGT GAC GGC AAA ATG AAA GAG C 3′ (For Primer), N6 - 5′ ATG AGG AGC GAG AAG AGG CTT GAC 3′ (Rev Primer).

[3] Probe for Light Cycler assay: Nucleocapsid LCR probe: 5′ LC Red 640 - ATTGGCACCCGCAATCC - phosphate 3′; Nucleocapsid Flu Probe: 5′—GAGCCTT GAATACACCCAAAGACC—fluorescein 3′.

[4] SARSNP fpr1/SARSNP rpr1/SARSNP prb1 Kuiken *et al.* 2003.

[5] SARSTM frp1/SARSTM rpr1/SARSTM prb1 Kuiken *et al.* 2003.

nested sub-genomic RNAs (sgRNA) sharing a common 3′-end. Genes encoded at the 3′-end are transcribed at high levels and represent the most abundant sgRNA species at least during infection in cell culture. Products of non-structural genes, such as the *RdRp* (*Pol*), responsible for replication and transcription of the viral genome, are needed in smaller amounts than structural genes, such as the NC protein involved in assembly of the virions. Consequently, sgRNA for the NC gene should be more abundant than sgRNA for the *Pol* gene in infected cells. This feature of coronavirus biology may be relevant for improving its detection in clinical practice. There are considerable differences in the concentration of viral RNA fragments in infected cells, with several log-fold increases in the amount of NC (mRNA) RNA in infected cells, compared with the transcripts of *Pol* genes (Thiel *et al.* 2003). This finding suggests that there may be some diagnostic advantages to targeting *NC* genes for molecular detection as well as other genes, to improve the overall sensitivity of detection, because the amount of viral template will be much higher, if clinical material contains virus infected cells as well as whole virus. Using clinical samples spiked with a mixture of SARS-CoV virus and infected cells, it is evident that detection of *NC* genes does provide some additional sensitivity (Table 8.1). Several laboratories have developed diagnostic PCRs for the detection of other regions of the genome, particularly the viral *NC* gene (Emery *et al.* 2004). This approach is consistent with the observation, that targeting the SARS-CoV NC region improved the sensitivity of detection more than a 100-fold in experimentally infected animals (Kuiken *et al.* 2003*a*).

8.6 Diagnostic developments

As might be expected in the first several months following the emergence of a new human pathogen, there has been an explosion of diagnostic developments, particularly in the commercial sector. One of the difficulties in validating new diagnostic tests is the availability of clinical material because over 90% of the cases worldwide occurred in Southeast Asia. It is likely that incremental gains in sensitivity of SARS-CoV PCR tests

will occur over the next few years as there is increasing use of Real-Time PCR platforms capable of detecting multiple targets and concurrent or multiplexing of SARS-specific and pan-corona tests. Greater gains in sensitivity may also come from techniques which concentrate on the biological sample prior to processing for nucleic acid extraction (Grant *et al.* 2003; Chan *et al.* 2004).

8.7 Virus propagation

It is fortunate that the SARS-CoV virus, in contrast to many animal coronaviruses, can be cultured easily in a variety of continuous cell lines, including FRhK and Vero E6 cells, produces a recognizable and distinct widespread cytopathic effect (CPE) (Fig. 8.3), and grows well at 33°C and 37°C. This has

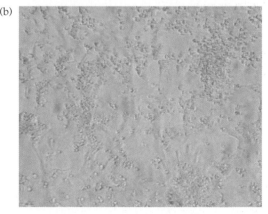

Figure 8.3 Mock infected Vero E6 cells (a) compared with cytopathic effect of SARS in Vero E6 cells (b) at 4 days post-infection.

(a)

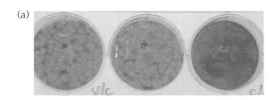

(b)

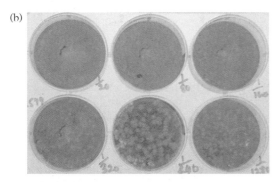

(c)

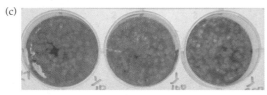

Figure 8.4 Neutralizing Antibody tests. Infectivity (a) and Plaque reduction assays (b,c) for the detection of SARS neutralizing antibodies. Virus infected cells are shown in the first two wells of panel A indicating clear plaque formation in Vero E6 cells 4 days post-inoculation, with mock infected cell control in the third well. Infection of virus in the presence of increasing dilution of SARS convalescent serum is shown in panel B and indicates total inhibition of virus growth at day 4 post inoculation with an IC50 serum titre of approximately 1/320. Non-SARS serum with no neutralizing activity is shown in Panel C.

allowed the recovery of infectious virus from affected individuals, which in turn expedited sequencing of the entire virus genome (Marra *et al.* 2003). Moreover, the development of infectivity assays has allowed quantification of virus infectivity and development of neutralization assays (Plaque reduction neutralization tests are shown in Fig. 8.4) Infectious virus has not been recovered beyond three weeks after illness onset even though virus is still detectable by RT- PCR for several days/weeks after this. The inability to detect infectious virus indicates the natural cessation of viral replication or the development of the antibody response (detectable from about day 10 post onset of illness) that may form complexes with virus, thereby affecting the ability to detect infectious particles.

8.8 Serological assays

As the virus produced a CPE in FRhK cells, virus infected cells were used as an antigen substrate before the aetiological agent had been described. Seroconversion using IF was the earliest serological test used to detect SARS (Peiris *et al.* 2003*a*). Use of IF indicated that seroconversion took place ca. 10 days after illness onset, but might not actually be evident in all cases until ca. 28 days after onset, as approximately 10–20% individuals did not have detectable antibodies until after day 21 (Peiris *et al.* 2003*b*). The late seroconversions noted may reflect the fact that many patients were treated with high dose steroids, which is likely to have delayed the antibody response, although this cannot be firmly concluded from the clinical datasets available. The only available laboratory method for excluding the diagnosis of SARS-CoV infection is to obtain a negative result on serological testing of a convalescent phase serum at 28 days after onset of symptoms. It is therefore essential for an understanding of the true disease burden to have robust and reliable serological tests.

The development of SARS ELISA tests followed rapidly after the identification of the virus, and the use of virally infected cells to prepare antigen for indirect ELISAs for the detection of SARS antibodies (IgM and IgG) has been possible because of the ability to culture virus to reasonable titre, and to use virus infected cells as a source of antigens (Fig. 8.5; Ksiazek *et al.* 2003; Kuiken *et al.* 2003*a*).

Analysis of antibody responses to SARS-CoV has so far shown limited cross reactivity with antibodies to human group 1 or group 2 coronaviruses. Although full evaluations are not complete yet and further data are required, some limited cross reactivity to group 1 animal coronaviruses has been noted (Ksiazek *et al.* 2003). The method of preparation of antigens and the formulation of serological tests may impact substantially on the ability to detect any cross reacting antibody. Understanding the impact of serological responses to other human coronaviruses on antibody response to SARS-CoV is important because it will affect the specificity of tests and conclusions about exposure to SARS-CoV in the absence of clinical illness. Serological data are developing

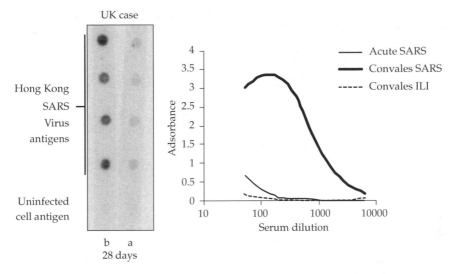

Figure 8.5 Detection of antibodies to SARS infected cell antigen by dot blot (Panel A(a,b)) and ELISA (Panel B). Sera from SARS positive UK probable case (Kuiken *et al.* 2003) at day 7 (a) Acute and day 28(b) Convalescent is shown in dot blot assay format indicating the detection of low levels of antibody early post-illness onset and seroconversion at day 28. Panel B. ELISA reactivity of serial dilutions of serum taken from (a) Acute SARS day 7 (b) day 28 Convalescent SARS (c) day 28 post-influenza A illness presenting with a clinical syndrome fulfilling the WHO case definition for 'Probable SARS'.

rapidly and early data suggest that high levels of neutralizing antibodies are formed following SARS infection and last for at least several months after infection. The use of neutralizing antibody tests (such as shown in Fig. 8.4) indicates that antibody to SARS may also cross neutralize related animal viruses, perhaps with a slightly lower titre and this is taken as a suggestion of more than one serogroup of SARS-CoV (Zheng *et al.* 2004).

The specificity of the SARS-CoV antibody response has allowed seroprevalence studies to be undertaken using IF, which have concluded that there was little spread of SARS-CoV in the general population in Hong Kong, based on blood donor screening (Donnelly *et al.* 2003). However, up to 40% of humans who are market traders of live animals or who are restaurant workers preparing, exotic meat of the putative wild animal reservoir (members of the Vivverid, Mustelid, and Canid families), showed evidence of exposure to SARS viruses, which has been taken to support the zoonotic origin of the SARS-CoV (Guan *et al.* 2003). Screening of archived healthy adult sera in Hong Kong (Zheng *et al.* 2004) taken before the SARS outbreak indicated that a small number had detectable antibody to the SARS-CoV, suggesting pre-existing evidence of exposure to a related virus.

One of the difficulties of screening individual sera, whether from cases of illness, for sero-surveillance or for contact tracing is the sensitivity and specificity of ELISAs or IF assays, which typically have sensitivities and specificities between 90% and 98%. This is true for almost all ELISAs used to screen human sera for many viral diseases, and usually leads to an algorithm of a screening assay followed by a confirmatory assay. Invariably, a small proportion of reactive sera will not be true positives after the first ELISAs. To improve the certainty of diagnosis, a serological strategy needs to be adopted, involving a second tier of tests (Fig. 8.6) with or without an additional second serum to test for seroconversion. Many laboratories have adopted a neutralization test as a 'gold standard' confirmatory assay, with typical neutralizing antibody titres of between several hundred and several thousand detectable at 28 days post onset of illness. The rise in neutralizing antibody may not exactly parallel the rise in total antibody detection, and may be somewhat slower to develop. However, tests which use virus-infected cells, or live virus, as required for whole-cell lysate ELISA assays, IF or neutralization tests require the growth of virus (Figs 8.4 and 8.5), which in turn requires a Biosafety Level 3 laboratory

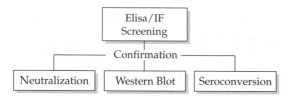

Figure 8.6 Suggested algorithm for serological testing of SARS.

and prevents the tests from being used widely. It is likely that trends in serological assay development will be towards the use of recombinant antigen ELISAs and finding surrogate methods for neutralization tests such as receptor binding assays which may be a safer alternative for the serological diagnosis of SARS. The limited data available internationally so far suggest good correlation between recombinant protein ELISAs, Western Blots, and IF results (Wu *et al.* 2004), but much more evaluation will be required to understand fully the relationships between antibodies and different coronaviruses.

There remains many unanswered questions about the nature of serological responses to infection with the SARS-CoV, despite the astonishing rapidity of development of robust diagnostic tests. The next few years will undoubtedly see the unravelling of the relationship between neutralizing and functional antibody and total antibodies to specific virus proteins, the duration and magnitude of antibody response in the context of disease protection, and a comparison of antibody response in children and adults. An attempt to understand serological relationships between different SARS-CoV viruses as well as between SARS-CoV and other human and non-human coronaviruses will benefit our understanding of the biology of coronaviruses as a whole, and assist in the understanding of the severity of SARS disease in humans. A very significant side effect of SARS related research is likely to be a greater focus on the burden of illness as a result of human coronaviruses and their role in acute respiratory and gastrointestinal infections, a neglected backwater of human virology.

Acknowledgements

The authors acknowledge the excellent technical work of the following members of the Health Protection Agency ERNVL laboratory staff, Ruth Reith, Jo Smith, Tracey Kesting, Ian Putwain, Victoria Gould, Carol Sadler, Brian Megson who assisted in the development of diagnostic tests for SARS in the United Kingdom, and the scientific support and advice of colleagues including Dr Robin Gopal, Dr Dhan Samuels, Dr Joanna Ellis, Dr Joanne Stockton, Pam Litton Judy Mitchell, and Dr Kirstin Edwards.

CHAPTER 9

Animal origins of SARS Coronavirus: possible links with the international trade in small carnivores

Diana J. Bell, Scott Roberton, and Paul R. Hunter

9.1 Summary

The search for animal host origins of severe acute respiratory syndrome coronavirus (SARS-CoV) has so far focussed on wildlife markets, restaurants, and farms within China. A significant proportion of this wildlife enters China through an expanding regional network of illegal, international wildlife trade. We present the case for extending the search for ancestral coronaviruses and their hosts across international borders into countries such as Vietnam and Lao PDR where the same guilds of species are found on sale in similar wildlife markets and food outlets. The three species which have so far been implicated, a Viverrid, a Mustelid and a Canid, are part of a large suite of small carnivores distributed across this region currently over-exploited by this international wildlife trade. A major lesson from SARS is that the underlying roots of newly emergent zoonotic diseases may lie in the parallel biodiversity crisis of massive species loss as a result of overexploitation of wild animal populations and the destruction of their natural habitats by increasing human populations. To address these dual threats to the long-term future of biodiversity, including man, requires a less anthropocentric and more inter-disciplinary approach to problems which require the combined research expertise of ecologists, conservation biologists, veterinarians, epidemiologists, virologists, as well as human health professionals.

9.2 Introduction

A World Health Assembly Resolution on 27 May 2003 recognized SARS as the first severe infectious disease to emerge in the twenty-first century which posed a serious threat to the stability and growth of economies and the livelihood of human populations. The causal coronavirus genome sequenced by Marra *et al.* (2003) defined a new fourth class of coronavirus subsequently referred to as SARS-CoV. Holmes and Enjuanes (2003) confirmed that the structure of the SARS-CoV genome suggested that it was neither a host-range mutant of a known coronavirus, nor a recombinant between known coronaviruses, and was unlikely to have been created by genetic engineering. Subsequent genetic analysis of isolates obtained throughout the 2002–3 epidemic by He *et al.* (2004) found that two genotypes predominated during the early phase of the epidemic in Guangdong Province. These viral genomic sequences were similar to those of coronaviruses infecting other mammalian hosts. However, during the second phase of the epidemic, which followed the first super-spreader event in Guangzhou, these authors found that SARS-CoV sequences contained a new 29 nucleotide deletion that dominated the viral population for the remainder of the epidemic (He *et al.* 2004). These latter findings indicate that the 2002–3 epidemic originated from a single source, consistent with the view that this source was animal.

The wildlife markets and restaurants in southern China became the focus of the search for SARS-CoV origins in April/May 2003. Joint teams of Chinese and World Health Organization (WHO) epidemiologists discovered that a number of the early SARS patients in Guangdong Province worked in jobs associated with the sale or preparation of wildlife for human consumption. On 23 May 2003, a team led by Yi Guan (University of Hong Kong) and colleagues from the Centre for Disease Control (CDC) Shenzhen, China announced at a press conference that they had isolated a coronavirus resembling SARS-CoV (identical apart from a 29 nucleotide base insert) from six (out of six) masked palm civets (*Paguma larvata*) and a raccoon dog (*Nyctereutes procyonoides*) in a market in Shenzhen, Guangdong Province, and that a third species present in the market, the Chinese ferret badger (*Melogale moschata*) elicited antibodies reacting against SARS-CoV (Guan *et al.* 2003). Some 25 individuals from eight of the many species sold for human consumption had been purchased for the investigation. The masked palm civets also seroconverted and their sera inhibited the growth of SARS-CoV isolated from humans. Five out of 10 civet dealers present in the market were found to have antibodies that cross-reacted with the SARS virus. Chinese authorities had responded by imposing a temporary ban on the hunting, sale, transportation, and export of all wild animals in Southern China and also quarantined all civets reared for human consumption in many civet farms across the area. A subsequent study found that prevalence of IgG antibody to SARS-CoV was significantly higher among animal traders than in a control population; 72 of 792 (13%) animal traders sampled in three animal markets in Guangdong Province tested positive for SARS-CoV IgG antibody compared to only 1–3% of people in three control groups (Yu *et al.* 2003). The prevalence of traders with IgG antibody varied between markets and was highest among those who reported trading primarily in masked palm civets (73%), wild pigs (57%), and muntjac deer (56%).

However, on 19 June 2003, Sun Qixin and colleagues at the Chinese Agriculture University (CAU) reported at a press conference that they had found no evidence of such viruses among their more extensive sampling of 54 wild and 11 domestic animal species collected from across six Chinese provinces. These samples had included 76 masked palm civets (three from Guangdong and a mix of 73 wild and farmed animals bought elsewhere) from which the CAU team isolated another coronavirus less similar to SARS-CoV (Normile and Enserink 2003). No further information on this quest was released until a brief announcement on 21 August 2003 following visits to markets and farms across Guangdong province by a joint team of 14 international specialists from the Chinese government, the WHO, and the Food and Agricultural Organization of the United Nations (FAO). This group reported finding SARS-like viruses in a range of vertebrate species including snakes, birds, and mammals and highlighted the urgent need for further serological testing of animals and humans and a strengthening of regulations in the farming, trading, and consumption of wildlife. In April 2004, Chinese newspapers reported that foxes, 'hedge-shrews' (species identity not clear from this translation), and 'cats' had been added to the list of SARS-CoV carriers and that 10.6% of 994 people working in animal markets in 16 cities across Guangdong Province carried 'positive antibodies' to SARS-CoV compared to only 3.25% of a sample of 123 people working in civet farms (ProMed). We still await the publication of this additional screening research but in the interim (August 2003) there were media reports that the above ban on the consumption of wildlife had been lifted by the Chinese authorities.

So far, this search for animal host sources has remained focussed on animal markets, wildlife restaurants, and farmed wildlife facilities within China. This chapter offers alternative perspectives on this search for the animal origins of SARS-CoV. First, we present the case for expanding this search in terms of both geographical area and range of species and products investigated, second we draw attention to recent ecological shifts in this region which favour the emergence of new zoonotic infections, and lastly we highlight the need for interdisciplinary collaboration with vertebrate and conservation biologists with specialist knowledge of potential host species and the international wildlife trade.

9.3 Geographical area of search

We believe that restricting the search for animal origins (wild or farmed) to within China may be flawed. A significant proportion of the wildlife sold in markets in southern China actually originates from neighbouring countries, reaching China through an expanding regional network of illegal wildlife trade. The existence of this extensive movement of animals highlights the need to extend the search for ancestral coronaviruses and their hosts across international boundaries into potential countries of origin of animals on sale in Guangdong (just 300 miles from Vietnam) where one finds the same guilds of species on sale in similar wildlife markets and restaurants.

In the past 5–10 years, Vietnam has become an important link in this international wildlife trade network and this trade has developed into an extensive illegal industry valued at over 20 million US dollars per annum. Some of the main trade routes for wildlife from the Lao People's Democratic Republic (PDR) and Vietnam are reproduced in Fig. 9.1.

In Vietnam, for example, the wildlife trade not only sources an expanding domestic market of wildlife meat restaurants, taxidermists, and traditional medicine shops within the country but the majority of species are also illegally exported to Chinese wildlife markets. This illegal export trade has been well documented for some years despite sustained efforts by Vietnam's National Forest Protection Department to control it. No accurate figures are available regarding the quantities of different species being shipped due to the illegal nature of the trade but turtles, civets, and other small carnivores, pangolins, snakes, tiger, and primates are among the species exported to China (Compton and Quang 1998; Roberton et al. 2004).

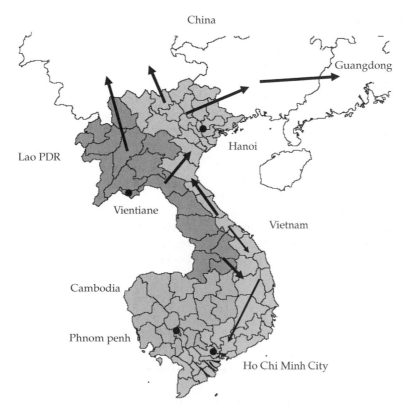

Figure 9.1 Some of the main wildlife trade routes in Southeast Asia and China.

Regular confiscations by Vietnamese Forest Protection Department rangers vary from a few individuals to truckloads. To illustrate the potential scale of demand within Vietnam alone, a recent survey in Vinh City, Nghe An Province, reported that about 600 kg of civet meat is consumed in just four wildlife meat restaurants per month, and volumes are expected to be far greater in Hanoi and other major cities of Vietnam. Although there were reports that the trade and consumption of small carnivores declined after their implication as a possible source of SARS-CoV (S. Roberton, personal observation), this decline was short-lived and civets soon reappeared in restaurants in both Hanoi and Da Nang. In Vietnam, increased demand from domestic and international markets together with rising market prices have escalated the level of criminal activities associated with this illegal wildlife trade (Roberton *et al.* 2003).

This widescale movement of possible host species within and across international borders through the wildlife trade raises a series of testable hypotheses concerning the geographical source and extent of the animal reservoir for SARS-like coronaviruses. It is possible, for example, that infective source animal(s) arrived at Guangdong markets and wildlife restaurants through illegal trade routes from newly exploited host populations in Lao PDR or Vietnam. Viral screening with generic probes of putative host species, plus parallel cohorts of human contacts, at different stages in this wildlife trade system is therefore required to determine whether such viral infections are endemic in wild host populations outside China (in Indochina and other Southeast Asian countries). An alternative hypothesis is that animals become infected at some point after entering the wildlife trade system, through mixing of species and/or populations which would not have contact in their native habitats. Such cross-infection could occur within the overcrowded conditions typical of wildlife markets across the region, where captured individuals of a range of traded reptile, avian, amphibian, and mammalian species have cross-exposure to each other, to rodent, avian, and invertebrate pest species moving freely within those markets (and food outlets) and to a series of human handler contacts (hunters, traders, cooks).

Ironically, those traded animals which survive the often protracted process of capture (typically snaring), handling, and long-distance journeys to wildlife markets and restaurants under covert conditions are likely to be the healthiest and most resilient individuals within captured cohorts.

The hypothesis that the source of SARS was a wild animal, possibly from outside China is supported by detailed analysis of the early epidemiology of the SARS epidemic in Guangdong (Xu *et al.* 2004). This latter study confirms that a high percentage (9 out of 23; 39%) of early cases (i.e. November 2002 to January 2003) were categorized as 'food handlers', that is, prepared and served food or handled, killed and sold animals for food, although none were livestock or poultry farmers. Also, it was more likely that early-phase patients (November 2002 to January 2003) lived close to a market selling and/or killing live animals than late-phase (February–April 2003) whereas 'living near a poultry or livestock farm or having other types of animal contact, including domestic pets or livestock, poultry, or specific wild animals or birds, was not associated with a high risk for SARS'. Of particular interest to the theme of this chapter was the observation that the index patient in Guangxi (the adjacent province) was a young man who worked as a driver for a wild animal dealer who 'supplied Guangdong market with wild animals from Guangxi, other Chinese provinces, and Vietnam'.

9.4 Range of potential host species and products

Published research (Guan *et al.* 2003) has so far implicated three species from three different families within the mammalian order Carnivora, as possible sources of SARS-like coronaviruses. These are the masked palm civet *P. larvata*, a viverrid, the Chinese (or large-toothed) ferret badger *Melogale moschata*, a mustelid, and the Raccoon dog *N. procyonoides*, a canid. However, these are just three of a large suite of small carnivores present across this geographical region. Other mustelids and viverrids known to occur in Vietnam and Lao PDR are listed in Table 9.1. There are 55 known species of mustelid in six sub-families

Table 9.1 List of Mustelid and Viverrid species found in Vietnam, Lao PDR, and China

Family	Sub-family	Genus	Species	Vernacular name	Vietnam	Lao PDR[a]	China	CITES
Mustelidae	Mustelinae	*Mustela*	*kathiah*	Yellow-bellied weasel	Y	Y	Y	App 3
			nivalis	Least weasel	Y	?	Y	
			strigidorsa	Stripe-backed weasel	Y	Y	Y	
			sibirica	Siberian weasel	Y	Y	Y	App 3
				Himalayan weasel				
		Martes	*flavigula*	Yellow-throated marten	Y	Y	Y	App 3
	Melinae	*Melogale*	*moschata*	Chinese ferret badger	Y	Y	N	
				Small-toothed ferret badger				
			personata	Large-toothed ferret badger	Y	Y	Y	
		Arctonyx	collaris	Hog badger	Y	Y	Y	
	Lutrinae	*Lutra*	*lutra*	Common otter	Y	Y	Y	App 1
				Eurasian otter				
			perspicillata	Smooth-coated otter	Y	Y	?	App 2
			sumatrana	Hairy-nosed otter	Y	?	N	App 2
		Aonyx	*cinerea*	Small-clawed otter	Y	Y	Y	App 2
				Oriental small-clawed otter				
Viverridae	Viverrinae	*Viverra*	*zibetha*	Large Indian civet	Y	Y	Y	
			Megaspila	Large spotted civet	Y	Y	?	
			tainguensis	Taynguyen civet	Y	?	?	
		Viverricula	*indica*	Small Indian civet	Y	Y	Y	
		Prionodon	*pardicolor*	Spotted Linsang	Y	Y	?	App 1
	Paradoxurinae	*Arctogalidia*	*trivirgata*	Small-toothed palm civet	Y	Y	Y	
				Three-striped palm civet				
		Paradoxurus	*hermaphroditus*	Common palm civet	Y	Y	Y	App 3
				Toddy Cat				
		Paguma	*larvata*	Masked palm civet	Y	Y	Y	App 3
		Arctictis	*binturong*	Binturong	Y	Y	Y	App 3
	Hemigalinae	*Chrotogale*	*owstoni*	Owston's Palm civet	Y	Y	Y	
		Cynogale	*lowei*	Lowe's otter civet	Y	?	?	App 2
	Herpestinae	*Herpestes*	*javanicus*	Small Asian Mongoose	Y	Y	Y	App 3
			urva	Crab-eating mongoose	Y	Y	Y	App 3

[a] The Lao People's Democratic Republic acceded to the Convention on International Trade in Endangered Species (CITES) from May 2004.

which include the badgers, otters, weasels, mink and polecats, martens, tayra and wolverine. Mustelids are distributed more widely than the Old World viverrids, occuring on all continents except Antarctica and Australia. Eleven of these 55 mustelids, representing three sub-families, are known in Vietnam (Roberton *et al.* 2003) and 10 of these are also reported to occur in Lao PDR (Duckworth *et al.* 1999). There are 36 known species of viverrids (civets and genets) classified into 20 genera within six sub-families; all are Old World species (Macdonald 2001). Eleven of these 36 viverrids, representing three sub-families, are known to occur in Vietnam including the recently

described Taynguyen civet (Sokolov *et al.* 1997). Nine of these are also known to occur in Lao PDR (Duckworth *et al.* 1999). The masked palm civet, common civet, and small Indian civet are the species most commonly found in wildlife restaurants across the region, but all nine species are eaten under the generic label of 'civet meat', depending on their availability.

Clearly, an ability to distinguish among these several species of small carnivores is an important pre-requisite in any search for possible hosts of SARS-like coronaviruses. Furthermore, the existence of this variety of closely related species within these two families of small carnivores highlights the need for comparative virological investigation of coronavirus evolution among closely related species of putative natural hosts. It is also worth noting that within the three sub-families of viverrids (civets and genets) represented across Indochina, there are a further 14 African species which are exploited within the African bushmeat trade (Schreiber *et al.* 1989). Again, comparative virological screening of this outgroup may be timely.

A common ecological characteristic of the three small carnivore species so far implicated (and indeed of those other carnivores, like cats and foxes, implicated in unconfirmed reports) is that their omnivorous diet may include small rodents. SARS-like coronaviruses have been isolated from rat populations recently sampled in southern China (Zhong 2004). This raises the possibility that small carnivores become carriers after exposure to infected rodent prey. A number of rodent species occur in this region. In Lao PDR, at least 28 species of murinae mice and rat species are known to occur, plus several rhyzomyine bamboo rat and platacanthomyine spiny and pygmy dormice species, prior to systematic rodents surveys in that country (Duckworth *et al.* 1999). In rural Lao PDR, these may be trapped for food in subsistence hunting and some sold on to urban food markets; some of these rodent species are also significant pests of agricultural crops.

It is worth noting that in Vietnam, the exploitation or trade in several of the small carnivore species such as the small Indian civet, striped-backed and yellow-bellied weasel is strictly prohibited under government legislation which recognizes their ecological importance as 'enemies of rats'. If rodents are the natural hosts of SARS-coronaviruses, widescale extermination of their natural small carnivore predators, could exacerbate rather than remove the problem. Comparative virological screening of the more frugivorous (e.g. binturong) versus the more carnivorous small carnivore species, may shed further light on the identity of the natural host species.

In common with a range of other species across this region, a number of these small carnivore species are now threatened with extinction as a result of overexploitation at unsustainable levels by an expanding international trade in wildlife.

Seven out of 11 viverrids and 5 out of 12 mustelids reported in Vietnam are listed as threatened in the 2000 Vietnam Red Data Book (the large spotted civet, the spotted linsang, the small-toothed palm civet, the binturong, Owston's palm civet, Lowe's otter civet, the Taynguyen civet, the least weasel, the Eurasian otter, hairy-nosed otter, smooth-coated otter, and the oriental small-clawed otter), while trade in 15 out of these 23 species is regulated under Vietnamese species protection legislation.

The status of populations in Lao PDR is largely unknown and/or difficult to assess, thus 6 out of 11 of the mustelids are listed as 'little known' and 4 as 'at risk' in Duckworth *et al.* (1999) and 4 out of 9 of the viverrids listed as 'at risk' or 'little known' in Lao PDR.

Although the primary end for most small carnivores which enter the wildlife trade is in wildlife restaurants in larger towns and cities, these animals are also exploited for other purposes across this region. Some enter private zoo collections or are kept as pets, the scent glands and body parts are used in 'traditional' medicines and perfumes, their skins sold for decoration, and civets specifically are used to produce weasel coffee. Roberton *et al.* (2003) report that civet penis is one of the wildlife products mixed with rice wine to produce a wildlife rice wine alleged to increase virility or libido in the consumer.

'Weasel coffee', one of the world's most expensive coffee beans, gains its unique qualities and flavour by being fed to captive civets and subsequently recovered from their excreta. In some Southeast Asian countries like Malaysia, the characteristic flavour and smell of weasel coffee and of the civet scent secreted by the perineal glands (present in all civet species) may be artificially manufactured, but in many areas these products are still recovered from captive civets. Given the high level of viral excretion of SARS-CoV reported in human patients (described by Peiris and Guan in Chapter 6, this volume) the possibility that any of these additional points of human to small carnivore contact could act as a source of cross-infection, merits investigation. Similarly, it may be useful to screen individuals (often with well-documented life-history details of age, origin, etc.) of these species held in zoos and other private collections around the world, for target coronaviruses.

9.5 Ecological shifts favouring emergence of new diseases

The IUCN (The World Conservation Union), Species Survival Commision (SSC) Action Plan for the conservation of viverrids and mustelids published 15 years ago highlighted habitat loss and fragmentation, particularly of tropical moist forests and wetland ecosystems, as the major threats to both families (Schreiber *et al.* 1989). That important collation of information on the status and conservation requirements of these small carnivore groups flagged the urgent need for population surveys and research into the ecological requirements of these little-studied species. The Action Plan also warned that 'the impact of hunting was growing with the rapid increase in human populations which results in a decrease in habitat quality and the fragmentation of Viverrid populations…and that this problem appeared to be greatest in the Upper Guinea rain forests and parts of Asia, such as China, Taiwan and Vietnam' (Schreiber *et al.* 1989, p. 14). The important point is that 20 years ago, even in Africa, while other 'more important' wildlife species were often sold by hunters at local markets, these small carnivore species tended to be consumed at home and were therefore regarded as opportunistically hunted subsistence food.

While the subsequent explosion in the African bushmeat trade has been well-documented (Hearn 2001; Barnes 2002; Fa *et al.* 2002, 2003, 2004; Bowen-Jones *et al.* 2003; Thibault and Blaney 2003), the depletion of wildlife in Asian forests has received less research attention (Bennett and Rao 2002). In Lao PDR, Duckworth *et al.* (1999) highlight wildlife as the second largest source of income after fish, for rural families, with a substantial increase in the overall trade in wildlife meat occurring in the late 1990s. They explain that the proportion of harvested wildlife sold, rather than consumed at home, is determined by a complex range of factors such as prevailing local economic situation, ethnic group, season, and accessibility to markets. While

more fish and aquatic invertebrates are eaten than all other vertebrate groups combined in lowland villages, forest mammals and birds are more important in upland villages away from water bodies (Foppes and Kethpanh 1997 cited in Duckwoth *et al.* 1999). Wildlife meat, which is usually sold as live animals in Lao PDR, is more expensive than that of domestic animals and is thus regarded as a luxury or health item (Srikosamatara *et al.* (1992). Duckworth *et al.* (1999) report that the only estimates of annual sales of wildlife in Vientiane's major market available, were those compiled by the former authors in 1992; attempts at tighter control of the wildlife trade during the 1990s had caused it to become clandestine and thus more difficult to quantify. The estimates reported in Srikosamatara *et al.* (1992) were 8000–10,000 mammals (of at least 23 species), 6000–7000 birds (over 33 species), and 3000–4000 reptiles (at least 8 species) at a value of 160,000 US dollars per annum and a total weight of 33,000 kg for that single market.

Duckworth *et al.* (1999) confirm that although much wildlife is consumed within Lao PDR, 'there is a massive illicit movement of live animals and parts of dead animals into neighbouring countries…A well-organised network in Vietnam takes wildlife, mostly alive, to China and much of this comes from Lao PDR'. While acknowledging that Lao wildlife had been traded for many years with other countries (e.g. rhino horn, ivory, animal bones), these authors cite increasing affluence in China and elsewhere in Southeast Asia, as fuelling the substantial increase in international wildlife trade over the previous 15 years. Certain Lao towns such as Ban Lak serve as important links in the supply chain to Vietnam and China and others, such as Ban Mai and Ban Singsamphan to Thailand (for wildlife from Lao PDR and Cambodia). At the end of the 1990s the major international threat to Lao wildlife was its use in traditional medicine, involving a range of species including tiger bones, turtles, civets, otters, primates, pangolins, snakes, and geckos; the number of species being moved to Vietnam for food or medicine far exceeded those shipped for pets or display (e.g. parakeets, hornbills, doves, and primates) (Duckworth *et al.* 1999).

Similar shifts and vast expansion in the hunting and trade of wildlife has occurred over this 15-year time period in Vietnam. Roberton *et al.* (2003), for example, describe how subsistence hunting has been replaced by sale into the wildlife trade for species such as civets, wild pig, deer, porcupine, and snakes and suggest that this has been driven by increased market prices and demand from emerging middle classes in larger towns and cities where government employees and businessmen form a major proportion of the wildlife restaurant customers.

In Vietnam, increased market value of wildlife has also led to increased sophistication of hunting techniques and criminal practices such as corruption, bribery, and associations with other forms of organized crime. International demand for wildlife, mainly from China, together with the above increased domestic demand within Vietnam has severely depleted populations such that hunting for certain species for the medicinal trade (e.g. tiger, bear, and pangolin) has shifted towards the forests in Lao PDR. Recent surveys of the wildlife trade by trained Vietnam's National Forest Protection Department rangers in Quang Nam Province, Vietnam found civets, snakes, wild pig, muntjac, sambar, turtles, porcupine, and pangolin to be the most heavily traded animal groups (Roberton *et al.* 2004). Seventy-four restaurants were found to be selling wildlife meat in that survey; wild pig, civet, porcupine, sambar, muntjac, and soft-shelled turtles were the most commonly consumed species, although small quantities of bamboo rats, squirrels, pangolin, small cats, serow, langur, and chevrotain were also sold. Up to 364 kg of civet meat was served monthly in just five restaurants and no differentiation was made between the species of civet sold.

The threat of significant biodiversity loss across this geographical region as a consequence of escalated levels of wildlife extraction and forest loss and fragmentation is clearly of major concern to conservation biologists (see below). However, this combination of events also has significant implications for human health since it presents a recipe of ecological conditions favourable for the emergence of new zoonotic diseases, including

SARS. These ecological shifts include:

(1) the change from subsistence hunting for local consumption to the sale of hunted animals into an expanding wildlife trade;

(2) the extensive cross-exposure within this wildlife trade of species and species populations which would not mix or contact under natural conditions (i.e. without human intervention);

(3) the exploitation of new source populations as areas become depleted of target species;

(4) their movement, often over vast distances, through an expanding international wildlife trade network; and

(5) to newly exposed human (or animal?) consumer populations.

9.6 Wildlife trade: a global threat to human health and biodiversity

Although man has hunted wildlife in tropical forests for at least 100,000 years, levels of exploitation have increased dramatically over recent decades to unsustainable levels across much of the humid tropics so that many of the species hunted are facing local or global extinction (Milner-Gulland *et al.* 2003). A common current misconception is that this 'bushmeat crisis' is unique to Africa but accelerated loss of forest species through overhunting first occurred in Asia, is currently occurring across Africa, and is predicted for South America over the next 10–20 years. This pattern mirrors that of the marked growth in human populations, forest loss, and development across these three continents (Milner-Gulland *et al.* 2003). Other factors contributing to dramatically increased levels of hunting include greater access due to forest fragmentation and road building, loss of traditional hunting controls, changes in hunting technology, and its increased commercialization, and long-distance transfer to urban markets where wild meat may be a preferred food (Robinson and Bennett 2000).

International conservation organizations have identified global biodiversity 'hotspots' which require highest priority conservation effort as a consequence of the high levels of species diversity and endemicity they contain and the high levels of threats they are currently experiencing. The geographical region highlighted above forms part of the Indochina region of the Indo-Burma biodiversity hotspot. This Indochina region appears among the top eight hotspots most likely to lose the majority of its animal and plant species as a consequence of continuing forest loss and species overexploitation at unsustainable levels (Davis *et al.* 1995; Dinerstein *et al.* 1999; Brooks *et al.* 2002; Anon 2004). The Indo-Burma region hotspot covers a land area of over 2 million sq. km and includes the majority of Vietnam, Lao PDR, Cambodia, Thailand, Myanmar, and an adjacent area of southwest China. This area incorporates enormous habitat and species diversity with high levels of endemism. In terms of mammals alone, this hotspot includes over 350 terrestrial species; approximately one quarter of these are endemic, that is, only found in this region of the world, and 70% of these endemic mammals are listed by IUCN as globally threatened (Brooks *et al.* 2002; Anon. 2004). Among this mammalian fauna, the discovery of a number of newly described species over the past decade, including three species of muntjac, the soala, and a new species of striped rabbit highlights the need for detailed faunal and floral surveys across the region (Dung *et al.* 1994; Giao *et al.* 1998; Timmins *et al.* 1998; Amato *et al.* 1999; Surridge *et al.* 1999; Matthee *et al.* 2004). The mammals considered at greatest risk as a consequence of illegal over-hunting for international wildlife trade, particularly with China, include all primates, pangolins, bears, cats, civets, Asian elephant, wild cattle, and deer (Anon 2004).

Globally, as well as posing a threat to biodiversity, the illegal wildlife trade poses a very real and serious risk to human public health. Many of the most dangerous infections to have been described have their origin in wild birds and mammals (Weiss 2001, reproduced in Table 2.1). This list includes some of the most feared infectious diseases ever to have affected human populations, for example, plague, smallpox, typhus, yellow fever, and AIDS. In some situations, the virus remains largely the same as that present in the evolutionary host species and multiple opportunities exist for spread from animals to humans. In other situations, the virus adapts itself to its new human host, becoming a human-specific

infection. In both these cases, there is considerable evidence that the resulting human infections frequently have enhanced virulence for their new human hosts (Osterhaus 2001). Against this background the illegal trade in wildlife can be seen as a real risk to human health. To re-emphasize this observation, the SARS epidemic was not the only disease associated with traded wildlife in 2003. There was also an outbreak of monkeypox in the United States associated with prairie dogs that had been in contact with Gambian Jumping rats imported from Africa in wildlife pet trade (Reed *et al.* 2004). Other recent outbreaks include ornithosis associated with a shipment of pet birds (Moroney *et al.* 1998) and an outbreak of *Salmonella* in the United Kingdom associated with imported terrapins (Lynch *et al.* 1999).

The trade in wildlife can also be a factor in the spread of infectious diseases to other domestic and wild animals as in the example of chytridiomycosis, an emerging disease of amphibians associated with the international restaurant trade (Mazzoni *et al.* 2003).

The size of the wildlife trade on a global scale is immense and is illustrated by the reports of (known) wild animal imports into the United States in 2002, namely over 38,000 live mammals, 365,000 live birds, 2 million live reptiles, 49 million live amphibians, and 216 million live fish (US Senate Committee Testimony on wildlife trade, 17 July 2003).

Action required to address this problem of species overexploitation in the wildlife trade is discussed in detail elsewhere (e.g. Milner-Gulland *et al.* 2003). For the Indochina region, the necessary actions proposed (Roberton *et al.* 2003) include:

(1) strengthen wildlife protection legislation;
(2) increase effectiveness of law enforcement activities;
(3) strengthen integrity of the National Forest Protection Departments;
(4) increase knowledge and monitoring of illegal activities;
(5) increase effectiveness of development interventions for biodiversity conservation;
(6) increase community participation in conservation;

(7) improve rescue, rehabilitation, and placement of animals confiscated from hunters and traders; **(8)** raise consumer awareness to reduce demand for wildlife meat and other products.

Current efforts to ban the sale and consumption of wildlife in China in response to its implication as the source of SARS-CoV, should be welcomed and fully supported by those with human health or biodiversity conservation as their primary concern. One of the major lessons from SARS is that the underlying root cause of newly emergent zoonotic diseases may lie in the parallel biodiversity crisis of massive species loss due to overexploitation of wild animal populations and the destruction of their natural habitats by increasing human populations. To address these dual threats to the long-term future of biodiversity, including man, requires a less anthropocentric and more interdisciplinary approach to problems which require the combined research expertise which includes ecologists, conservation biologists, veterinarians, epidemiologists, virologists, as well as human health professionals.

CHAPTER 10

Epidemiology, transmission dynamics, and control of SARS: the 2002–2003 epidemic

Roy M. Anderson, Christophe Fraser, Azra C. Ghani, Christl A. Donnelly, Steven Riley, Neil M. Ferguson, Gabriel M. Leung, Tai H. Lam, and Anthony J. Hedley

10.1 Summary

This chapter reviews current understanding of the epidemiology, transmission dynamics, and control of the aetiological agent of severe acute respiratory syndrome (SARS). We present analyses of data on key parameters and distributions and discuss the processes of data capture, analysis, and public health policy formulation during the SARS epidemic. The low transmissibility of the virus, combined with the onset of peak infectiousness following the onset of clinical symptoms of disease, transpired to make simple public health measures, such as isolating patients and quarantining their contacts, very effective in the control of the SARS epidemic. We conclude that we were lucky this time round, but may not be so with the next epidemic outbreak of a novel aetiological agent. We present analyses that help further understanding of what intervention measures are likely to work best with infectious agents of defined biological and epidemiological properties. These lessons learnt from the SARS experience are presented in an epidemiological and public health context.

10.2 Introduction

The re-emergence of the viral aetiological agent of SARS in China at the end of 2003 (Paterson 2004), following the epidemic earlier in the year affecting many countries, rang alarm bells in the WHO and elsewhere. Thankfully, prompt action by the Chinese authorities in the isolation of suspect cases and in instigating contact tracing and quarantine measures served to effectively contain the virus. By the end of February 2004, only three confirmed cases and one probable case had been reported with no chains of onward transmission identified (WHO 2004*b*). Where the virus re-emerged from remains uncertain, but the prime suspect as an animal reservoir host remains the civet cat (Paguma larvata), and the foci for spread from this host to humans seem to be the animal markets in China, especially those in Guangzhou, in the Guangdong province (Webster 2004). Guangdong province is where the major 2003 outbreak originated that infected more than 8000 people and killed 774 (He *et al.* 2004). One measure introduced by the Chinese authorities, following the re-emergence of SARS late in 2003, was a large cull of the civet cat populations in the animal markets and breeding farms, estimated to have involved the removal of over 10,000 animals (Watts 2004). Molecular epidemiological studies suggest that the coronavirus in humans is very closely related to a strain found in civet cats, but differs slightly from the one that caused such devastation earlier in 2003. A clear priority is further surveillance of animals in settings where the human virus spread extensively so as to better understand the origins of the epidemic in humans and the role of animal reservoirs. In the global response to the 2003 SARS epidemic, orchestrated by the WHO, there were five priority tasks at the start of the outbreak. These were the identification of the aetiological agent of the new disease SARS, the development of diagnostic tests to detect the virus, the development and assessment of treatment protocols to reduce morbidity and mortality, estimation of the key epidemiological parameters that affected spread and persistence, and the formulation and implementation of appropriate public health interventions. Most of these tasks were completed rapidly, including the identification of the viral aetiological agent (Drosten *et al.* 2003; Ksiazek *et al.* 2003; Peiris *et al.* 2003c), the delineation of the full genome sequence of the virus (Marra *et al.* 2003), the evaluation of key epidemiological parameters (Donnelly *et al.* 2003), and the impact of different interventions (Lipsitch *et al.* 2003; Riley *et al.* 2003). Problems remain, however, in the areas of quick and accurate diagnosis and effective therapeutic interventions. Detection of the presence of the virus soon after onset of clinical symptoms remains difficult, with the most sophisticated RT–PCR tests still providing only limited sensitivity following the onset of fever. Sensitivity can be improved if samples from the lower respiratory tract can be obtained in the second week following the onset of clinical symptoms. Serological tests are highly sensitive, but after only 21 days following clinical onset (Li G. *et al.* 2003). With respect to clinical interventions to reduce morbidity and mortality, as yet too little has been done to date to merge clinical patient databases from different settings and countries so as to provide sufficient power to perform rigorous evaluations, taking account of the many confounding factors such as age and various co-morbidities. In any such analyses, a note must be taken of differences among countries in the way clinical symptoms were recorded. This chapter reviews current understanding of the key epidemiological determinants of the transmission dynamics of SARS-CoV, and evaluates what interventions worked best in different settings, using mathematical models to give structure and clarity to the analysis. We also consider gaps in current

knowledge and priorities for future research to improve predictions of observed pattern and the evaluation of the impact of interventions for novel infectious agents.

10.3 Data needs for epidemiological study

The study of the transmission dynamics of an infectious agent is typically based on simple or complex mathematical frameworks (Anderson and May 1991). The goals in model formulation and analysis can be many and varied. They include delineating what needs to be measured to better understand observed pattern, identifying the key determinants of this pattern, and evaluating how different interventions introduced at various stages of the epidemic influence the future incidence of infection and associated disease. For a new pathogen the first of these goals is of central importance both in guiding data collection and analysis, and in the formulation of policies to protect public health. The following sections describe the key steps in data collection and analysis, with the aim of providing robust estimates of the key parameters (and their distributions) that influence transmission and control. Much between-patient variability is often associated with the parameters that influence the typical course of infection in a patient and transmission. Thus, the full distributions must be estimated so that variability in properties such as the incubation period of the disease, the infectious period and how infectiousness changes over time following infection, times from onset of clinical symptoms to isolation in a healthcare setting, and times from isolation to recovery or death are fully understood.

10.4 The construction of a patient database

The creation of a patient database that integrates socio-demographic detail with clinical information, such as treatment and outcome, and epidemiological data, such as contact tracing information and behavioural questionnaire data, is central to the real-time analysis and control of infectious disease outbreaks. Ideally, the electronic database should have one central point of control (such as in a government department or designated research centre), be web-based with password protection for remote data entry, and be designed to act as a registry and monitoring system to inform policy formulation and allow analyses to be updated daily throughout the epidemic. All patients suspected of having contracted SARS within a country or administrative region should be entered into this database with a unique patient-identifying code. Appropriate measures should be taken to protect patient identity and to conform to data protection legislation. At a global level, such countrywide data should ideally be shared with the WHO, either in its entirety or in a pared down form which includes case incidence over time and basic epidemiological and clinical information, to inform their policy formulation and advisory notices. Few countries achieved such real-time collection and synthesis of information during the SARS outbreak. Arguably, the best example of good practice occurred in the Hong Kong Special Administrative Region of China, where the Health, Welfare, and Food Bureau of the government (in collaboration with university-based public health professionals), created a system called SARSID (SARS Integrated Database) to collect and collate case information. Even in this setting, however, problems were encountered in linking case information with clinical treatment data held in healthcare settings, and with the results of contact tracing which were held in a separate database managed by the police service. In many countries, the appropriate databases and associated analyses were fully assembled and completed only after the end of the epidemic. As a consequence of the SARS experience (and experiences with other rapidly developing infectious disease outbreaks; see Ferguson *et al.* 2001*a,b*), the development of appropriate software and the training of personnel to use it should be a priority for all government health departments.

10.5 Case definition and clinical symptoms

The case definition of SARS has changed since the emergence of the 2002–3 epidemic. However, the following definition developed by the WHO was used throughout the main period of spread in 2003 (www.who.int/csr/sars/casedefinition/en/). Two criteria were used in this definition. The first definition included a person presenting after 1 November 2002 with history of high fever (greater than 38°C) and cough or breathing difficulty, and one or more exposures during the 10 days prior to onset of symptoms. Exposures are defined as close contact (having cared for, lived with, or had direct contact with respiratory secretions or body fluids) with a person who is a suspect or probable case of SARS; history of travel to an area with recent local transmission of SARS; or residing in an area with recent local transmission of SARS. The second definition included a person with an unexplained acute respiratory illness resulting in death after 1 November 2002, but on whom no autopsy had been performed and who had one or more exposures during the 10 days prior to onset of symptoms. A probable case was defined by the WHO to have three criteria as follows: (1) a suspect case with radiographic evidence of infiltrates consistent with pneumonia or RDS on chest X-ray; (2) a suspect case of SARS that is positive for SARS-CoV by one or more assays; and (3) a suspect case with autopsy findings consistent with the pathology of RDS without an identifiable cause. Because all SARS diagnoses were based on exclusion of other possible causes (e.g. influenza), a case could be excluded if an alternative diagnosis was made at a later stage following admission to hospital. Throughout the first epidemic and over the months since its termination on 5 July 2003, many cases have been reclassified on the basis of information from virological assays or serological tests based on sera drawn from patients after cessation of clinical symptoms. Clinical symptoms at admission to hospital, and during hospital stays for confirmed SARS cases (based on virological confirmation) have been recorded in various studies (see Donnelly *et al.* 2003; Tsang *et al.* 2003). At admission, high fever, malaise, cough, and headache seem to be the most common symptoms. For confirmed SARS cases, high and prolonged fever and diarrhoea are typical symptoms. Virus can be isolated from sputum, urine, and faeces during the mid-to late clinical phase of symptoms (Peiris *et al.* 2003*c*).

10.6 Incubation period

The incubation period is defined as the time from infection to onset of clinical symptoms of disease. This duration is often influenced by factors such as the infecting dose of the virus, the host genetic background, the route of exposure, and the age of the patient. The determination of the form of this distribution and its summary statistics at the start of an epidemic of a novel infectious agent are of great importance, given their significance to the duration of quarantine and to contact tracing. The average incubation period also influences the time-scale of the development of the epidemic, by its influence on the rate at which secondary cases are generated. Infection events cannot be observed, but data on patients with short and well-defined periods of exposure to known SARS cases can be used to estimate the distribution of the incubation period. Estimation of the incubation period is based on sets of patients with a short

exposure period of known date to a suspect SARS case. This information may be collated via contact tracing or from questionnaires. The estimates for SARS are based on about 200 cases from five regions that experienced moderate to severe epidemics (Hong Kong, Mainland China (Beijing and Guangdong), Taiwan, Singapore, and Canada). The data are summarized in Table 10.1. Donnelly *et al.* (2003) report a mean of 6.37 days (subsequently revised to 4.6 days after the end of the epidemic), with about 95% of all estimates lying between 2 and 12 days. An observed distribution based on 70 cases in Guangdong and Beijing is shown in Fig. 10.1(a). Figure 10.1(b) shows the best-fitting gamma distribution to 86 cases with short exposure intervals from Hong Kong.

10.7 Time from onset of clinical symptoms to admission to hospital

Very early on in the SARS epidemic it was understood that reducing the time from onset of clinical symptoms to admission to hospital and subsequent isolation was an important measure to reduce the net rate of transmission within a community or country (Donnelly *et al.* 2003). Most countries compiled statistics on this distribution, with Hong Kong, Taiwan, and mainland China having access to such information as the epidemic progressed. Onset and admission times are both

Table 10.1 Incubation period of SARS

Country/region	Mean (days)	Number of cases	Reference
Hong Kong	4.6	81	Leung *et al.* (2004*a*)
Mainland China	4	70	WHO (2003*f*)
Singapore	5.3	46	WHO (2003*f*)
Canada	5	42	Varia *et al.* (2003)

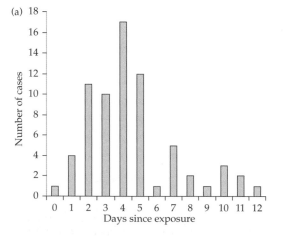
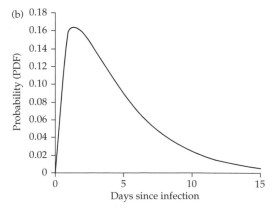

Figure 10.1 Incubation period distribution of SARS in (a) 70 cases in Quangdong (mean, 4.5 days) and (b) 86 cases in Hong Kong (mean, 4.6 days), where exposure was known to have occurred over a short interval of time (Donnelly *et al.* 2003).

observable events. However, in the early phase of a new epidemic, analyses must allow for censoring as a result of incomplete observation. If censoring is not taken into account, the distribution will be biased towards short onset-to-admission times, because patients are only eligible to be included in the hospital-based database on admission to hospital. Patients with recent onsets and long onset-to-admission times are less likely to have been admitted to hospital and thus to be included in any analysis. One such distribution, compiled following the cessation of the epidemic to eliminate the problem of censoring, is recorded in Fig. 10.2(a). As a consequence of public health announcements using the press and media, many regions managed to encourage individuals with symptoms of severe respiratory tract infection to report rapidly to hospitals. For example, in Hong Kong, the mean period shortened greatly over the course of the epidemic (Fig. 10.2(b)).

10.8 Time from admission to hospital to discharge

The duration of stay in hospital for those who recovered was typically long, with a mean of approximately 25 days in Hong Kong. Longer durations of stay were associated with older patient age and the presence of co-morbidities. The duration of hospital stay is an important statistic for the effective management of a SARS outbreak, because it describes one aspect of hospital resource use. Ideally, while admitted, patients should be cared for in isolation facilities with the application of rigorous infection control measures.

10.9 Time from admission to death

SARS is a very pathogenic disease with a high case fatality rate (CFR). The time periods from admission to death are again of importance to health care planners in terms of resource use within the

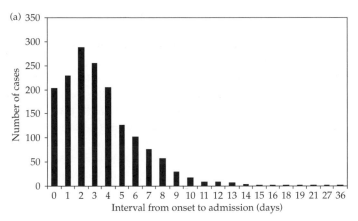

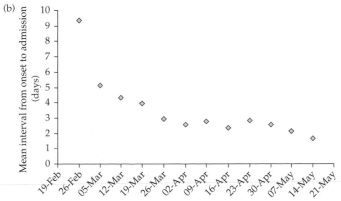

Figure 10.2 Distribution of interval from onset of clinical symptoms to admission to hospital in Hong Kong. (a) Overall distribution; (b) mean interval plotted by week of onset of symptoms.

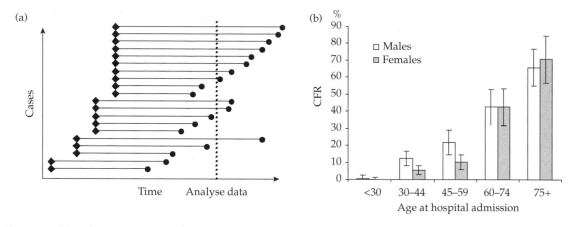

Figure 10.3 (a) A schematic representation of right-hand tail censoring, where estimation underestimates the magnitude of mortality unless account is taken of cases in which the outcome is not known at a defined point in time (t_m). This problem typically arises in the early stage of an epidemic when there are many patients remaining in hospital for whom the final outcome (death or recovery) is not known. (Donnelly *et al.* 2003). (b) The final SARS CFR in Hong Kong stratified by gender (white bars, males; grey bars, females) and age at hospital admission.

Table 10.2 Summary of the means of four key distributions based on data from Hong Kong (see Donnelly *et al.* 2003)

T_1: Exposure-to-onset (incubation period): mean = 4.6 days, variance 15.9 days². 95% of infected individuals onset within 12.5 days. Analysis based on interval-censored exposure data.

T_2: Onset-to-admission: reflects rapidity of diagnosis and hence isolation. Decreased from an average of 4.9 days early in epidemic to less than 2 days by mid May.

Admission-to-death (for patients who died)—mean of 35.9 days.

Admission-to-discharge (for patients who recovered)—mean of 23.5 days.

hospital setting. In the Hong Kong setting the mean time was 36 days but with a high variance. Age and other co-morbidities greatly increased the mortality rate (Leung *et al.* 2004*a*). This long period generates difficulties in the estimation of the CFR unless methods account for the censoring of data before outcomes are fully known (see Fig. 10.3). A summary of the key distributions derived from data from Hong Kong is presented in Table 10.2.

10.10 Case fatality rates

The term CFR is widely used to describe the proportion of those who acquire an infection that eventually die from the disease induced by the aetiological agent. The CFR is not strictly a rate: it

is a simple proportion or percentage. The first published study of case fatality in a sample of SARS patients for which outcome was known, or adjusted for by appropriate statistical methods for censoring of the data (Fig. 10.3(a)), was that of Donnelly *et al.* (2003). Using a modified Kaplan–Meier-like non-parametric method this study gave estimates of 6.8% for patients younger than 60 years and 55% for patients older than 60 years. At the end of the first epidemic of SARS-CoV it is possible to examine the mortality associated with the disease in more detail. Overall, a WHO summary suggests a global average of about 15%. However, this figure hides much variation: there was little mortality in the young and high levels in the elderly. Multivariate analyses identify age effects and the presence of co-morbidities (such as pre-existing heart or respiratory tract disease) as the most important determinants of the outcome (Leung *et al.* 2004*a*). Figure 10.3(b) shows age- and gender-specific estimates of the CFR from 1628 patients from Hong Kong. Similar patterns have been recorded in Singapore and Taiwan. Lower rates were reported from mainland China (Beijing and Guangdong) but no detail is available as yet concerning laboratory confirmation of reported SARS cases and how these fatality rates relate to patient age and co-morbidity. In most studies laboratory testing has now become an integral part of mortality assessment to ensure that a reported SARS case, based on clinical features, is confirmed by either virus isolation or serology following recovery.

10.11 Infectious period

A key determinant of the pattern of spread of an infectious agent is the infectiousness distribution, both before and after the onset of clinical symptoms. Two approaches to estimation of the time course of infectiousness within a typical patient are the study of secondary case generation and the measurement of viral load given the assumption that this is proportional to infectiousness through contacts. For SARS-CoV the efficiency of transmission to close contacts appears to be greatest from patients with overt clinical symptoms, usually during the second week following onset. A study reported at the WHO meeting in Geneva in May 2003 but not yet published based on cases in Singapore suggests that peak infectiousness as judged by the generation of secondary cases is about days 7–8 following onset of clinical symptoms. The main conclusion of these analyses is in good agreement with a study by Peiris *et al.* (2003c) of changes over time in viral load (in nasopharyngeal aspirates and nose or throat swabs) following the onset of clinical symptoms of SARS-CoV in 329 patients from Hong Kong. In this study quantitative RT–PCR was used to

determine viral shedding. Maximum virus excretion from the respiratory tract occurs on day 10 of illness and declines thereafter to a low level at day 23. Virus in stools seems to start later than in respiratory excretions, with peak between days 12 and 14 and a slower decline thereafter. These results are summarized in Fig. 10.4. Virus can also be detected in urine, indicating wide organ involvement in pathogenesis (WHO 2003f). Retrospective quantitative studies of viral shedding in patients following recovery and discharge from hospital, based on collected samples of respiratory

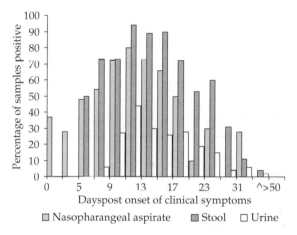

Figure 10.4 Studies of viral shedding in SARS patients on various days following the onset of clinical symptoms, in stool (dark-grey bars), urine (white bars), and nasopharangeal aspirate (light-grey bars) (Peiris *et al.* 2003c).

Infection	R_0	Percentage transmission that must be blocked to prevent epidemic
SARS	2–3	50–67%
HIV	2–5	50–80%
Smallpox	5–10	80–90%
Pandemic influenza	5–25	80–97.5%

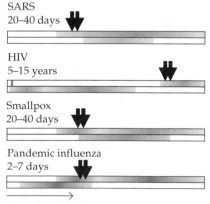

Figure 10.5 Key descriptors of infection for SARS and some infectious diseases. Right, schematic representation of the incubation and infectious distributions, plus when isolation of patients might occur on the basis of onset of clinical symptoms that result in diagnosis (Fraser *et al.* 2004). For each infection, the upper bar represents infectiousness while the lower bar represents intensity of symptoms as a function of time since infection. Patient isolation is represented by large arrows. The bars are labelled by an overall time since infection

tract excretions, faeces, and urine, are currently underway in a number of countries. For the study of transmission dynamics, quantitative measurements are of great importance to define a distribution of infectiousness before and after onset of clinical symptoms. The viral shedding studies that are available to date suggest that transmission could occur via close contact involving respiratory tract excretions, and via faecal or urine contamination of surfaces. A schematic representation of the relationship between the average incubation and infectiousness periods is presented in Fig. 10.5.

10.12 Atypical presentation of SARS and asymptomatic infection

Atypical presentation of SARS has been documented in a number of papers, where symptoms have included fever and diarrhoea, sometimes with bloody stools, but with no respiratory symptoms (e.g. Hsu *et al.* 2003; Chow *et al.* 2004). The incubation periods in such patients ranged from 3 to 8 days, and transmission on to contacts was observed, especially in hospital settings. Such

observations might suggest that the recorded cases of SARS, based on clinical criteria, may underestimate the extent of transmission and hence estimates of the case reproductive number, R_0 (Fig. 10.6; Lipsitch *et al.* 2003; Riley *et al.* 2003). Further observations relating to the distribution of cases by age, matched with the known age distribution of given populations, revealed a deficit of cases in the young and an excess in the elderly. This pattern could arise from frequent asymptomatic infection in the young and more severe infection in the elderly (Fig. 10.7). After the end of the epidemic, a number of studies have been undertaken to assess the extent of transmission from index cases, where no formal identification of SARS was made in such contacts. Serological surveys, for example, have been carried out in Hong Kong using contact tracing data to identify known contacts of SARS cases, to assess the degree of seropositivity in contacts with no recorded symptoms of SARS. In one study of over 1000 serum samples taken from over 3000 contacts of recorded SARS cases, only 0.3% were positive for SARS-CoV immunoglobulin-G antibodies (Leung

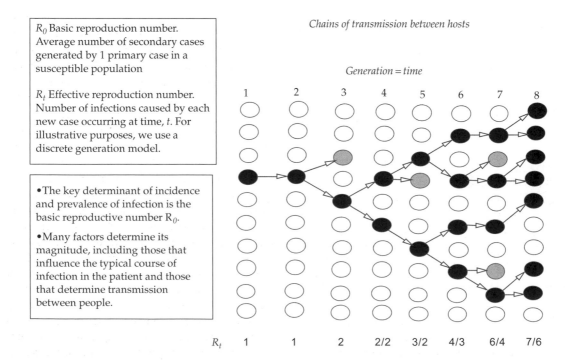

Figure 10.6 Diagrammatic representation of chains of transmission. The speed of spread is determined by the case reproductive number R_0.

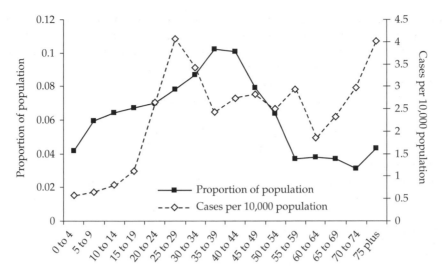

Figure 10.7 Age distribution of 1628 reported SARS cases and population age distribution in Hong Kong.

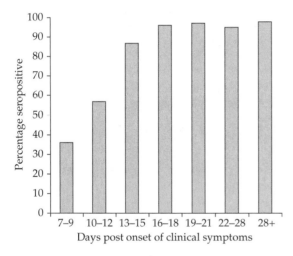

Source	No. samples	No. positive	% positive
Clinics	777	10	1.3
Hospitals	620	49	7.9
Total	1397	59	4.2

Figure 10.8 Serological studies of SARS patients and contacts with SARS patients in Hong Kong hospital and clinic settings (Li G. *et al.* 2003). Seroconversion in most patients occurs some 16–18 days after the onset of clinical symptoms, while contacts with such patients by hospital and clinic staff resulted in around a 4% seroconversion rate in individuals who were not diagnosed with SARS.

et al. 2004*b*). This result is reassuring, and goes some way to dispelling the doubt that recorded clinical cases of SARS reflect only a small proportion of transmission events. In hospital settings a higher fraction of contacts (who were largely hospital staff) were subsequently found to be seropositive (Fig. 10.8).

10.13 Super-spreading events

The epidemics of SARS-CoV in different countries with a moderate to large number of cases were characterized by a few super-spreading events (SSEs), where one case generated large numbers of secondary cases (Fig. 10.9). It is important to note that these events were most probably created by different combinations of person-related characteristics (e.g. high viral shedding) and environmental factors (e.g. contamination by fomites or close contact in a healthcare setting). The occurrence of such events created a distribution of secondary case generation with a high variance and concomitantly a long right-hand tail. Those in the tail of this distribution played a very important role in the emergence of the epidemic and its spread from country to country. One of these events occurred in a hotel in Hong Kong, where an ill traveller from Guangdong infected many other hotel residents, resulting in transmission to many countries from this single case. Others occurred in a hospital setting in Hong Kong, an air flight from Hong Kong to Beijing and in healthcare settings in Beijing, Singapore, and Toronto (Shen *et al.* 2004).

A detailed study of the event in a Beijing hospital revealed that one patient with 74 close contacts generated 33 secondary cases. These secondary cases generated a further 43 cases before this chain of transmission petered out (Shen *et al.* 2004).

Evidence from Guangdong province in China, during the very early stages of the global epidemic, suggests that most cases seem to have occurred in food handlers (individuals who kill, handle, and sell animals and meat, and those who prepare and serve food) (Breiman *et al.* 2003; WHO 2003*f*). Following this initial stage, the primary mode of person-to-person transmission appears to be via direct contact with respiratory droplets and exposure to fomites in settings where close contact

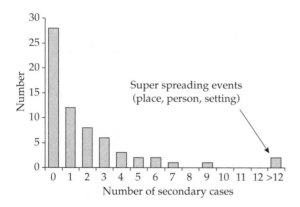

Figure 10.9 Schematic representation of the distribution of secondary cases. For SARS, most index cases generated none or a few secondary cases (with an average of ca. 2–3), while a few generated many.

occurred either in a household or a healthcare facility. In the total epidemic worldwide about 21% of recorded cases were in healthcare workers (WHO 2003). Other transmission events occurred in the general population (often unknown in nature) either in workplaces, taxis, or aeroplanes. The localized nature of transmission in defined environments suggests an agent of low transmissibility that requires close contact, either with an ill patient or with a recently contaminated surface. There is no direct evidence of faecal–oral transmission but the high and persistent viral shedding in faeces suggests that this could be a route of significance. The exact route of transmission is always difficult to determine and the relative importance of respiratory, faecal, and urine excretions remains unclear at present. For the purposes of the analysis of the transmission dynamics of the virus, the most important factors are the settings in which transmission occurs, the incubation and infectious periods, and the distribution of secondary cases.

10.14 Epidemic growth

In regions with significant number of cases, such as Hong Kong, Taiwan, mainland China, and Singapore, the typical pattern of epidemic growth was an initial period of stuttering chains of transmission, interspersed with one or two major SSEs. This was followed by a period of exponential growth slowing to reach a peak and then a period

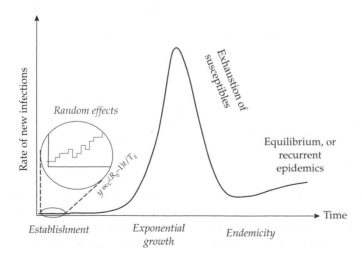

Figure 10.10 Schematic representation of the phases of epidemic growth after the introduction of an infectious disease into a virgin population. In the early phase of growth the rate of increase of cases is exponential with growth coefficient $(R_0 - 1)t/T_g$, where R_0 is the case reproductive number and T_g is the average generation time (Anderson and May 1991).

of steady decline with perhaps one or more SSEs leading to temporary resurgence, before the epidemic decayed with a cessation in chains of transmission (Fig. 10.10). The decay phases were of varying durations, depending on the efficacy of the interventions introduced in the different regions. The epidemic in mainland China had two phases, with initial spread in Guangdong province followed by a major epidemic in Beijing.

10.15 Transmission dynamics

Mathematical models of the transmission dynamics of infectious agents are valuable tools in making assessments of both what needs to be measured to understand spread better and what interventions used alone or in combination are most likely to be effective. They provide a template within which to integrate epidemiological and biological data. In the early- to mid-stages of the SARS epidemic, a number of research groups formulated mathematical models of viral spread of varying complexity. At one end were the simple deterministic susceptible–infected recovered frameworks (SIR) (Lipsitch *et al.* 2003), and at the other were more complex stochastic frameworks with more accurate description of disease progression and some representation of spatial structure, SSEs, and mixing (Riley *et al.* 2003). Approaches of intermediate complexity were also adopted (Lloyd-Smith *et al.* 2003).

The chain of transmission events within an epidemic is an expanding one if each primary case, on average, generates more than one secondary case. The average number of secondary cases generated in a susceptible population is termed the basic reproductive number, R_0 (Fig. 10.6). As the epidemic develops, the effective reproductive number at time t, R_t, which describes the generation of secondary cases in a partly susceptible population, decreases and eventually settles to unity if the disease becomes endemic. The pattern of epidemic growth is governed by two factors: the number of secondary cases generated by one primary case at the start of the epidemic, R_0, and the average time taken for the secondary cases to be infected by a primary case, termed the generation time or serial interval, and denoted as T_g (Anderson and May

1991). Essentially, R_0 determines how intensive a policy will need to be to control the epidemic, whereas both T_g and R_0 determine the time available to implement suitably intensive controls. For diseases that are highly infectious with short incubation periods, such as measles ($R_0 > 17$, $T_g < 11$ days), population-wide control requires the long-term reduction of the recruitment of susceptible people, through widespread childhood immunization. By contrast, for less infectious agents (R_0 ca. 2–10) that have longer incubation periods ($T_g > 20$ days), if an outbreak is detected in its earliest stages, there is sufficient time for localized control measures to be successfully applied (Fig. 10.5). One aim in model development for SARS spread in defined regions was therefore the estimation of both the basic reproductive number and the generation time to assess how difficult it might be to bring the epidemic under control.

Longitudinal monitoring of the magnitude of a further parameter, the effective reproductive number at time t, R_t, also provides crucial information on the success of the interventions that have been implemented to date. For an epidemic to be under control the magnitude of R_t must be less than unity: each primary case generates on average less than one secondary case such that chains of transmission stutter to extinction.

What is the best method to estimate R_0 in an emerging crisis? One simple approach is to estimate the doubling time of the epidemic, t_d, in its early stages, taking account of the stochastic fluctuations that typically occur in the early stages of any epidemic's development (Anderson and May 1991). Estimation of the key parameter, R_0, can be achieved by fitting an exponential growth equation. For simple epidemics of a directly transmitted respiratory or gastrointestinal pathogen, during early growth in a totally susceptible population, the doubling time t_d is related to the magnitude of R_0 by the simple expression

$$t_d = (\ln 2)D/(R_0 - 1),$$

where D is the average duration of the latent plus infectious periods (essentially the generation time T_g; Fig. 10.10). In the absence of knowledge of D, a range of assumptions will have to be made for its value, to get some idea of the magnitude of R_0 (Anderson and May 1991). In the early stages of the SARS epidemic, contact tracing data, especially that based on SSEs, suggested that the value of t_d was somewhere between one and a few weeks (Galvani *et al.* 2003). This method was used by Lipsitch *et al.* (2003) to estimate R_0 based on choosing a few time-points from several separate epidemics. The method was adjusted to allow for a skewed distribution of secondary infections, which amounted to treating SSEs as extreme points from a continuous distribution.

However, the approach based on doubling times is not very robust. Better non-parametric approaches to estimate R_0 directly from time-series can be based on either examining the ratio of incidence to prevalence, or on estimating the likelihood of any person having infected any other. Both approaches are based on the estimated distribution of generation times (Wallinga and Teunis 2004). The latter approach can be complemented by contact tracing data. The disadvantages are that it does not disaggregate different contributions to R_0 and it is purely descriptive of the data. Another method is to fit a mathematical model of the transmission dynamics of the infectious disease. Although robust, this approach is very parametric, in the sense of being dependent on making a

good choice for the framework of the model to fit the known biology and epidemiology.

The simplest models are based on the classification of the population into various disease states such as susceptible, infected but not yet infectious (latent), infectious, and recovered or dead. Equations for each state were constructed denoting rates of flow between the states. These rates may be represented as constants (with an exponential waiting time distribution for movement between states) or by distributed variables given availability of appropriate data (model structures with realistic distributions were used in Riley *et al.* (2003) and Lloyd-Smith *et al.* (2003); see Fig. 10.2). For SARS, the simplest structure is represented in Fig. 10.11, which depicts in a flow chart an additional class to those outlined above to reflect isolation or quarantine, such that a patient is infectious but unable to transmit. Such models may be stratified by factors such as age, spatial location, or environmental setting (i.e. within a healthcare setting), and may be formulated within a deterministic or stochastic framework.

Population heterogeneity ideally needs to be accounted for, reflecting, for example, variation in infection risk with spatial location, variation in

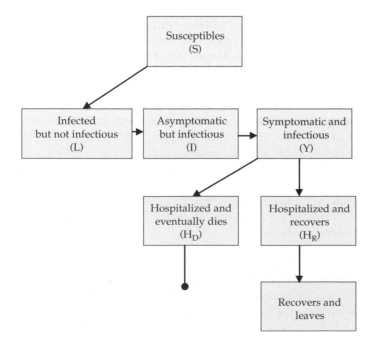

Figure 10.11 Compartmental framework for a stochastic model of the transmission dynamics of the viral aetiological agent of SARS (Riley *et al.* 2003).

contact rates between groups, and between-case variability in infectiousness (see Fig. 10.9; Riley *et al.* 2003). Heterogeneity in R_t between cases appears to be particularly important for SARS because of the occurrence of SSEs. These are defined as rare events where, in a particular setting, an individual may generate many more than the average number of secondary cases. To what extent SSEs are simply extreme values in skewed distributions of infection events (resulting from heterogeneous contact rates) or whether these are special events created by particular settings or host plus virus genetic backgrounds, is uncertain. Some insight can be gained by examining the SIR model with homogeneous mixing: in this case the distribution of secondary infections for each index case is already skewed, given by a geometric distribution with mean R_0 and variance $R_0(R_0 + 1)$ rather than the intuitively expected Poisson distribution with mean and variance of R_0 (Ferguson *et al.* 2004). The geometric distribution provides an adequate fit to the observed distribution of secondary infections (see Fig. 10.9). The probability of one individual infecting n_c or more people is then

$$p(n \geq n_c) = (1 - 1/R_0)^{n_c}.$$

Allowing for heterogeneous contact patterns does not usually greatly change this result. The Hong Kong epidemic, for example, was characterized by two large clusters of cases, together with ongoing transmission to close contacts. In the first cluster, at least 125 people were infected on or soon after 3 March in the Prince of Wales Hospital by the index patient for the Hong Kong epidemic (Lee, N. *et al.* 2003). In the second cluster, an unknown number of people were infected from a probable environmental source in the Amoy Gardens estate (Kwung Tong district). Following mixing with fellow residents, families, and friends, over 300 people became infected. Examination of local reports of SARS investigations supports the distinction between these two large SSEs and the other contact-based infections, where many occurred in a hospital setting. Furthermore, our simple analysis, taking the highest range of R_0 values of 5, results in the probability of generating 125 or more secondary infections being $p(n \geq 125) < 10^{-12}$, that is, the probability of such a large cluster arising even once by chance is

very, very small. It may be that the distinction between typical infection events and SSEs reflects the two different routes of transmission so far identified as likely for this virus, namely respiratory exudates and faecal–oral contact. However, much still remains uncertain about possible routes of transmission in these SSE settings.

Choice of a suitable model framework must be governed by the degree to which the investigator wishes to capture varying degrees of heterogeneity. A variety of approaches are possible, ranging from a simple deterministic compartmental approach with mixing between patches or settings, to a spatially explicit, individual-based stochastic simulation structure. Riley *et al.* (2003) adopted a stochastic, metapopulation compartmental model, given the quality of the data available in real time from the Hong Kong region. A metapopulation approach was considered to be appropriate because the incidence of SARS varied substantially by geographical districts in Hong Kong. A stochastic model was employed because chance fluctuations in case numbers can be large in the early stages of an epidemic. Stochastic models predict both average trends and variability, so that a more robust assessment can be made to examine what changes are likely to be caused by chance and what changes genuinely reflect process and the impact of interventions. They classified the population of each district of Hong Kong into susceptible, latent, infectious, hospitalized, recovered, and dead individuals. Data were available to characterize the distributions around these transitions from one compartment to the next. Epidemiological coupling between districts was assumed to depend on their adjacency. Incubating and infectious categories were further divided into multiple stages, chosen in number and duration so as to match accurately the estimated delay distributions determining disease progression and diagnosis (Fig. 10.2; Donnelly *et al.* 2003; Riley *et al.* 2003). Multiple realizations of the stochastic model were performed, both for parameter estimation and to generate predicted case incidence time series. The mean time from the onset of symptoms until hospital admission and subsequent isolation of suspect SARS cases reduced significantly over the course of the epidemic. Changes in the onset-to-hospitalization distribution were treated as an input to the model.

Riley *et al.* (2003) assumed that infectiousness began just before the onset of symptoms and remained constant during the symptomatic phase. With hindsight this was a reasonable assumption. More sophisticated assumptions could now be made given knowledge of how infectiousness changes before and after clinical onset (Peiris *et al.* 2003c; Fig. 10.4). Simulations were seeded explicitly with the Prince of Wales Hospital and Amoy Gardens clusters. Model fit to the observed case-incidence data in Hong Kong was qualitatively good, both in terms of capturing the temporal development of overall incidence and the pattern of spatial spread (Fig. 10.12). Fitting the model to observed trends provided estimates of both R_0, temporal changes in R_t, and the generation time T_g (Riley *et al.* 2003), and as such this approach has many advantages over the use of simpler model constructs given good availability of data in real time. Because the model was seeded explicitly with the two large SSEs, the estimate of R_0 measures the contribution of all non-SSE transmission, including community and hospital transmissions. The contribution of SSEs to R_0 can be calculated only heuristically, but this does not imply that the contribution was unimportant. Indeed, it is possible to construct a hypothetical scenario where the community and hospital contribution to R_0 are below unity, but where

SSEs push R_0 above this critical threshold. This would have led to extended periods of epidemic decay between SSEs, until case numbers by chance became sufficient that SSEs began chaining together, causing large and rapid epidemic growth.

The disadvantages of using a more sophisticated and statistically robust approach to estimating R_0 is the need for good computational facilities as well as good data. The development of reliable and efficient parameter estimation methods that do not rely on brute computational force should be a priority.

Estimates for R_0 were based on various methods and on data for a variety of regions. The estimates were in good agreement, despite the different methods employed and the various epidemics in different regions, with an average value of approximately three, independent of setting (Table 10.3). It is important to note that these estimates are based on case reports of individuals with overt clinical symptoms that lead to an initial diagnosis of SARS. To date, however, there are no confirmed cases of transmission from asymptomatic individuals (WHO 2003f). The main conclusion to be drawn from these estimates of R_0 is that SARS-CoV is of low transmissibility in comparison with other directly transmitted viruses such as influenza A (R_0 of about 7 or more) and the measles virus (R_0 of about 15–18 prior to widescale immunization (Anderson and May 1991)). Further confirmation of this low level of transmissibility is provided by analyses of SARS cases within those placed in quarantine as a result of close contact (either in healthcare, family, work, or transport settings) with a suspect SARS case. In Taiwan, for example, out of 131 to 132 people placed in quarantine, only 45 were recorded as probable SARS cases (Lee, M. L. *et al.* 2003).

The factors that triggered SSEs remain poorly understood at present. The causes probably

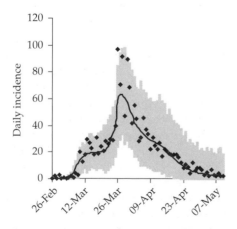

Figure 10.12 The SARS epidemic in Hong Kong and the fit of a multi-compartment meta-population stochastic model (from Riley *et al.* 2003). The dots are reported SARS cases and the solid line is the best fit model. The vertical grey bars denote 95% prediction intervals.

Table 10.3 Estimates of the basic reproductive number, R_0

Reference	Region	R_0	Comments
Riley *et al.* (2003)	Hong Kong	2–3	Excluding SSEs
Lipsitch *et al.* (2003)	Canada and Singapore	3	
Wallinga and Teunis (2004)	Singapore	3.3	

involve both environmental factors and determinants of the infectiousness of the index patient (the amount of virus excreted in respiratory tract exudates, faeces, and urine, and the duration of shedding). The importance of environmental factors is well illustrated by the high proportion of infections worldwide that occurred in healthcare settings (about 21% of all reported SARS cases (WHO 2003f)). In the estimation of R_0 it is important to recognize that this key epidemiological parameter is a mean drawn from a distribution with high variance. Those events in the right-hand tail of the distribution of secondary case generation may or may not constitute a separate class generated by distinct environmental or case infectiousness factors (Fig. 10.9).

10.16 How was the epidemic brought under control?

To evaluate how different control interventions might impact on any given epidemic during its emergence and early growth, we ideally need to use a mathematical model of transmission that embeds estimates of transmission efficiency and the details concerning the typical course of infection, to explore both what works best and in what combination, and the degree to which a specific intervention must be applied. For example, in the case of SARS, obvious questions are how important is it to reduce the time between onset of clinical symptoms to isolation or quarantine within a healthcare setting, and what time interval should be the target (i.e. within 1 or 2 days). For international and governmental agencies, the questions may be more complex, such as the value of introducing travel restrictions to and from affected areas, and the effectiveness of screening of passengers at airports for elevated temperature. Such measures may be costly to introduce and may have grave economic consequences for affected regions. It is therefore highly desirable to have available some sort of quantitative template to allow assessments to be made during the heat of the crisis.

For SARS the options for intervention within a country were limited to public health measures, in the absence of a vaccine or effective therapies.

There are essentially six intervention categories, namely: (1) restrictions on entry to the country and screening at the point of arrival for fever; (2) isolation of suspect cases; (3) the encouragement of rapid reporting to a healthcare setting following the onset of defined clinical symptoms, with subsequent isolation; (4) rigorous infection control measures in healthcare settings; (5) restrictions on movements within a country (restricting travel, limiting congregations such as attendance at school); and (6) contact tracing and isolation of contacts. To study in quantitative terms their respective impacts on transmission or the impacts of different combinations applied with varying efficiencies, each category must be captured within the mathematical model. One simple illustration is given in the flow chart in Fig. 10.11, where a category denoting infectious but isolated is represented. Interventions may reduce the magnitude of R_t but fail to reduce its value to less than unity. In these circumstances the incidence of new infections declines, as if the epidemic is waning, but in reality the trend is towards a new endemic state with the infection still persisting. During a crisis, it is difficult to interpret correctly whether or not changes in incidence following the introduction of control measures indicate (1) decay to probable extinction or (2) continued transmission but at a reduced rate. It is in these circumstances that mathematical models can play an important role as a template for the repeated estimation of R_t through time. Once R_t drops below unity, and stays there, the epidemic is under control provided no relaxation in implementation of the introduced interventions takes place. During the Hong Kong outbreak in 2003, combinations of reductions in onset to hospitalization, in population contact rates (mixing) and with healthcare setting transmission (improved infection control procedures) reduced the effective reproductive number to about 1.0 by 21 March, 0.9 by 26 March, and then to 0.14 by 10 April (Riley $et\ al.$ 2003).

Teasing out the relative contributions of different interventions is more difficult to achieve if the only quantitative outcome measure is cases of disease reported each day. Ideally other data are available such as changes in travel patterns, the decay in the interval between disease onset and isolation, and the fraction of all contacts of a suspect case traced within a defined time interval. For SARS, aside from case numbers, very few data were available day by day during the course of the epidemic in any given setting, except for information on the temporal change in the distribution of times between onset and isolation (see Table 10.2). Various attempts have been made to dissect the differing impacts of various interventions but with limited success to date. Some of these analyses were based on fitting models to case data to estimate parameters reflecting the efficacy of defined controls (Riley *et al.* 2003), whereas others are more abstract in the sense that parameter values were changed within a model and conclusions were drawn on model predicted trends (Lipsitch *et al.* 2003; Lloyd-Smith *et al.* 2003). Conclusions drawn from both approaches depend on model structure and parameter assignments, and as such should be accepted with caution.

Pooling the results from the published analyses (largely from Lipsitch *et al.* 2003; Lloyd-Smith *et al.* 2003; and Riley *et al.* 2003), the following conclusions can be drawn. Isolation and quarantine, contact tracing, improved infection control procedures, and self-imposed movement and mixing restrictions that limited contact were very effective in combination. They induced the dramatic changes in R_t after the peaks in the epidemic in all regions that were badly affected. Reductions in the onset to admission times were important in most settings owing to the late onset of infectiousness after onset of symptoms of disease. High impact can also be attributed to changes in contact rates (mixing) and better infection control plus isolation and quarantine of symptomatic patients in hospital settings. Spatially explicit models also suggest that restriction on movement between locations within defined communities could have played a useful role in limiting spread. Transmission in most regions was highly localized.

To date, detailed model-based analyses of the effectiveness of contact tracing for SARS suggest that it was far less effective than commonly perceived. More retrospective analyses are required in this area, using large contact tracing databases. A similarly urgent priority is analysis of the effectiveness of travel directives. Preliminary unpub-

lished studies suggest that they were effective in restricting between-country spread. However, this conclusion remains to be confirmed by detailed analyses of travel patterns between major cities before, during, and after the SARS epidemic.

Global success in the control of SARS was partly a result of certain epidemiological and biological characteristics of the infectious agent. In the absence of effective vaccines or treatment, understanding the factors that make containment of SARS feasible is important for evaluating how best to control future outbreaks of newly evolved pathogens. Two public health policy options exist for controlling the spread of a novel directly transmitted infectious disease agent: (1) effective isolation of symptomatic individuals (which includes rapid hospitalization after the onset of clinical symptoms) and (2) tracing and quarantining of the contacts of symptomatic cases. Both measures rely on rapid dissemination of information to facilitate accurate diagnosis of the symptoms of the disease.

For SARS, the timing of the onset of symptoms relative to peak infectivity is probably the most crucial factor in the success of simple public health interventions aimed at reducing transmission. In SARS patients, peak viraemia appears to occur between 5 and 10 days after the onset of symptoms (Peiris *et al.* 2003c). Although viraemia does not always predict infectivity, the very low levels measured in the days immediately after the onset of symptoms suggest that peak infectivity occurs somewhat later. Also, no confirmed cases of transmission from asymptomatic patients have been reported to date in detailed epidemiological analyses of clusters of SARS cases (Ksiazek *et al.* 2003; Lee, N. *et al.* 2003). This suggests that for SARS there is a period after symptoms develop during which people can be isolated before their infectiousness increases. It is during this period that transmission can be very effectively interrupted by isolation and quarantine. The second feature is the low transmissibility of SARS-CoV, with its moderately low basic reproductive number, with the exception of the settings in which SSEs occurred.

A recent study (Fraser *et al.* 2004) attempts to analyse why SARS was so effectively contained, using a generic mathematical model for directly transmitted agents. The approach adopted is comparative, and centres on the definition of two key properties of transmission and the typical course of infection, R_0, and the proportion of the area under the viral load curve in a typical patient that occurs prior to the onset of easily diagnosable symptoms. They show that the proportion of infections that arise prior to the onset of symptoms (or via asymptomatic infection), termed θ, is as strong a predictor of success of the simple public health control measures as the inherent transmissibility of the aetiological agent as measured by R_0. Isolation of a proportion ε of symptomatic individuals can control an outbreak if the following expression is satisfied:

$$\varepsilon > (1 - 1/R_0)/(1 - \theta),$$

which can never be reached when $\theta R_0 > 1$. Drawing crisp conclusions is more difficult in the case of contact tracing, or some combination of isolation and contact tracing. In these circumstances a combination of approximate analytical methods and individual-based simulation studies are required to gain insights (Fig. 10.13).

From published studies, Fraser *et al.* (2004) estimate these quantities (R_0 and θ) for two moderately transmissible viruses, SARS-CoV and human immunodeficiency virus 1 (HIV $-$ 1), and for two highly transmissible viruses, smallpox and pandemic influenza A. They conclude that SARS and

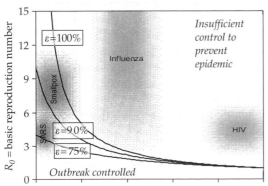

$\theta =$ Proportion of infections that occur prior to symptoms or by asymptomatic infection

Figure 10.13 Estimates of R_0 and θ for four infectious diseases, and the potential impact of patient isolation performed with varying degrees of efficacy ε; (Fraser *et al.* 2004).

smallpox are easier to control using these simple public health measures. This study therefore suggests that in an emerging epidemic of a novel agent, both clinical epidemiological studies of pathogen load and clinical symptoms, plus contact tracing to assess when transmission occurs during the typical course of infection, should be a priority.

10.17 Discussion

The evolution, spread, and persistence of infectious diseases are facilitated by the mobility of contemporary society, for example, through air travel, the continued growth in the world population, and the steady rise in the number of densely crowded urban areas (the so-called mega-cities with populations of over 10 million people), especially in Asia. As such, epidemic outbreaks of novel infectious agents are likely to become more common in the twenty-first century than in any previous period of human history. We therefore need to be prepared, and the 'SARS' experience provided many lessons for the future.

What are the lessons to be learnt from the SARS epidemic with respect to the detection and control of novel infectious agents? As an initial task it is important to find the agent that is the cause of observed morbidity and mortality and then to establish whether or not the agent is novel. Careful pathological, microbiological, and virological study is the key to discovery of the aetiological agent. With current sequence data on known pathogens, the problem of novelty is relatively easy to solve. The SARS epidemic showed clearly how effective international collaboration (and competition) resulted in the whole genome sequence of the SARS-CoV being available early in the epidemic. In the not too distant future, whole pathogen genome sequencing will be routine in most laboratories in developed countries. Difficulties remain in the poorer regions of the world, with limited surveillance and inadequate laboratory expertise. It is of particular importance in the most populous countries of the world; namely, China, India, and Indonesia (Anon 2004a). It is clearly in everyone's interest to greatly enhance global surveillance capabilities, especially in developing regions, and concomitantly to improve basic training in infectious disease and molecular epidemiology.

Effective surveillance structures aim to detect unusual clusters of morbidity and mortality in space and time. What constitutes such a cluster requires robust statistical analysis, and a time history of what normally occurs, taking account of seasonal and longer-term dynamical cycles and chance fluctuations in disease incidence (Anderson and May 1991). It is not too difficult to imagine that in the near future, automated software will be put in place in the richer regions of the world (such as North America and western Europe, which have good data capture systems for infectious disease reports) to analyse reported data on a daily basis to alert authorities of such unusual spatial and temporal clusters. However, it should be noted that the alert physician at the point of contact with sick patients who recognizes an unusual pattern of morbidity and mortality is the foundation of good infectious disease surveillance.

A related problem concerns whether or not the nascent epidemic is indeed about to expand, with R_0 in excess of unity. Several recent studies have started to address this question, taking account of the fact that even if R_0 is less than unity, some long chains of onward transmission will arise by chance before the epidemic stutters to extinction. The key statistics are the average cluster size and the average length of the transmission chains. Statistical and simulation tools are being developed to try and help in such assessments (Ferguson et al. 2004), and have been applied recently in the analysis of human cases of bird flu resulting from the major H5N1 epidemic in birds in Asia in the early part of 2004. Detailed contact tracing and clinical investigation could be used early in an outbreak to determine θ, the proportion of infections that occur prior to the expression of symptoms, and thus the likely impact of simple isolation and quarantine measures (see Fraser et al. 2004).

More generally, after the surveillance and detection problem, the next set of issues concern data capture, the development of diagnostic tests and treatment algorithms, and the identification of public health measures to control epidemic spread. Real-time data capture and associated analysis to reveal how the epidemic is expanding and how interventions are acting to slow down the pace of spread is essential. Few countries or regions did well on this front during the SARS epidemic, and the WHO struggled to collate detailed data in a timely manner from the affected countries. More must be done in Asia, Europe, North America, and the WHO, to improve the information feed into a 'command and control' centre for epidemic outbreak analysis and control. As some countries learnt to their cost, not having a clear command and control structure to manage an outbreak can delay the decision-making process. One central authority needs to collate and analyse data on a day-by-day basis. Furthermore, someone at this centre needs to have the authority to ensure that regional centres and healthcare settings submit data in a timely manner and that the best available scientific advice forms the basis for policy formulation. A section of this chapter describes experiences in Hong Kong where the health authorities performed well in this context in the mid-to late-phase of the epidemic.

Deciding well before an outbreak emerges what needs to be collected and what sort of analyses should be done day by day is an obvious starting point in the preparation for future outbreaks. Unique patient identifiers should be used to record all socio-demographic, clinical treatment, and epidemiological information (including contact tracing where the nature of contacts and the time period over which they are sought is well defined). Careful thought is needed to define data fields and apply effective data capture across all healthcare settings. Web-based, password-protected systems need to be ready to be put into action, with information fed daily to one centralized database for analysis and interpretation. No one country or region had such a system in place prior to the emergence of SARS. Ideally some common database and software structure should be used across all countries and regions, such that the WHO could capture information relevant for the global management of an outbreak.

Contact tracing and monitoring travel at points of entry and exit are part of this data capture process. The speedy and accurate collection of contact tracing data serves many purposes. First it acts as a public health measure, in the sense that it gives an opportunity to isolate or quarantine those in close contact with a suspect case. Equally important, however, is the fact that it provides a source of information to estimate key parameters and distributions, and modes of transmission. The incubation period is one key parameter, as are estimates of the distribution, and mean of the effective reproductive number. In most settings that were badly affected by SARS, the percentage of contacts traced within a few days was very limited. We need to learn more about how best to do such tracing for directly transmitted agents, and how best to analyse and interpret the data given uncertain denominators.

The effectiveness of temperature screening at points of entry and exit as a control measure to limit between-country transmission is uncertain at present. This needs more detailed retrospective analysis, as does the controversial measure of travel directives issued by the WHO at various stages of the epidemic. These almost certainly induced substantial changes in business and leisure travel patterns, and had a major impact on the economies of badly affected regions such as Hong Kong, mainland China, Taiwan, Singapore, and Ontario in Canada. More research is needed to establish clear guidelines for the circumstances under which such directives should be issued by the WHO.

The development of rapid diagnostic tests available at the point of patient contact is a clear priority in managing new outbreaks. The particular biology and pathogenesis of SARS-CoV made this task difficult to accomplish during the early- and mid-phases of the epidemic. Much has been learnt in this context, and the sharing of materials, reagents, and viral isolates orchestrated by the WHO was an encouraging aspect of the SARS experience.

A further lesson concerns the topics of clinical epidemiology and treatment algorithms. As noted earlier in this chapter, a key property that influences the likelihood of successful control is the typical relationship between the onset of clinical symptoms and viral load as a surrogate marker of infectiousness. With some notable exceptions (Peiris *et al.* 2003*c*), not enough attention was paid to quantifying these properties day by day for large samples of patients. Furthermore, the devel-

opment of effective treatment algorithms to reduce morbidity and mortality was delayed by poor sharing of patient information. With small numbers of patients in the early stages of a new epidemic, pooling of clinical data in an international database is essential. Randomized clinical trials cannot be conducted easily in the heat of a crisis, and hence careful analysis of observational databases with sufficient patient records to deal with confounders such as age and pre-existing comorbidities is the only way to decide which pattern of patient management and treatment is most effective.

With respect to the issue of data analysis and the design of the most effective intervention measures for pathogens with specific biological and epidemiological properties, a clear need is the development of generic mathematical models for a wide variety of pathogen types (including vector-transmitted viruses), with differing biological and transmission properties. More than one type of model is needed to deal with problems at a local level (perhaps even within a healthcare setting), at a community scale and within an international context. Prior exploration of what control option or combination of options works best in defined situations is a clear priority. One approach is that adopted by Fraser *et al.* (2004), but other model templates and methods of analysis would be highly desirable, using more sophisticated stochastic individual-based models. We need to understand more clearly how different interventions impact on agents with given properties, particularly if it is possible to put such measures in a cost-effectiveness framework. The issues of travel directives and airport screening for fever immediately come to mind. We understand very little at present about how effective they were in limiting the spread of SARS-CoV. More important, however, is the issue of isolation, containment, and contact tracing. Analyses by Fraser *et al.* (2004) provide a starting point for deciding whether such simple public health tools will work effectively if applied with a given efficacy, to control the spread of specific pathogens with defined biological and epidemiological properties (Fig. 10.13). Mathematical models also provide a framework within which different intervention strategies can be evaluated during the course of an epidemic (see Ferguson *et al.* 2001*a,b*). Estimation day by day of the effective reproductive number R_t (the average rate of generating secondary cases) provides a quantitative measure of success or failure.

The SARS epidemic caused much suffering, significant mortality, great disruption to social and work activities, and considerable economic losses. Draconian public health measures involving the isolation and quarantining of hundreds of thousands of people, and tight restrictions on travel, had to be put in place in some countries. However, it was brought under control—and relatively quickly—with the WHO playing a vital role in coordinating the international response. The quick and effective response of the WHO to the SARS crisis did much to restore faith among the many critics of the effectiveness of international agencies with large bureaucracies and limited resources for action. But it is difficult to escape the conclusion that the world community was very lucky this time round, given the very low transmissibility of the agent, plus the fact that fairly draconian public health measures could be put in place with great efficiency in Asian regions where the epidemic originated. Given the litigious nature of people in North America in particular, and to a lesser degree in western Europe, the control of SSEs in these regions might have presented greater problems if mass quarantining had been required. In the next global epidemic of a directly transmitted short-generation-period infectious agent we may not be so lucky, either in terms of the biology of the agent or the region of its origin. Thus one of the major dangers arising from the effective control of SARS is complacency. Sentiments of the type 'we have been successful once—we will be again' may be far from the truth. Simple public health measures worked well for SARS, but the persistence of the virus (or its close relatives) in animal reservoirs means that re-emergence will occur, as seen at the end of 2003 and the early part of 2004. However, the continuing threat from SARS needs to be kept in perspective, given that influenza A causes many tens of thousands of deaths annually in developed countries. Many informed observers feel that the real threat in the future is an antigenically novel influenza virus, of both high pathogenicity and transmissibility. In these circumstances, simple public health measures are unlikely to be effective (see Fig. 10.13), and other options such as more draconian movement restrictions, the greater availability of antiviral drugs, and expanded vaccine development and production facilities, will be needed to prevent a devastating impact.

CHAPTER 11

Dynamics of modern epidemics

Dirk Brockmann, Lars Hufnagel, and Theo Geisel

11.1 Summary

The application of mathematical modelling to the spread of epidemics has a long history and was initiated by Daniel Bernoulli's work on the effect of cow-pox inoculation on the spread of smallpox in 1760 (Bernoulli 1760). While most studies concentrate on the temporal development of diseases and epidemics, their geographical spread is less well understood. The key question and difficulty is how to include spatial heterogeneities and to quantify the dispersal of individuals (Keeling *et al.* 2001; Smith *et al.* 2002; Keeling *et al.* 2003; Lipsitch *et al.* 2003). In a well established class of models spatial dispersal is accounted for by ordinary diffusion (Murray 1993). This approach admits a description in terms of reaction-diffusion equations which generically exhibit epidemic wavefronts propagating at constant speeds. These wave fronts were observed for instance in the geotemporal spread of the Black Death in Europe from 1347–50 (Langer 1964; Noble 1974; Mollison 1991; Grenfell *et al.* 2001). However, today's volume, speed, and non-locality of human travel (Fig. 11.1) and the rapid worldwide spread of severe acute respiratory syndrome (SARS) (Fig. 11.2) demonstrate that modern epidemics cannot be accounted for by local diffusion models, which are only applicable as long as the mean distance travelled by individuals is small compared to the geographical scope of the model.

In this chapter, we focus on mechanisms of the worldwide spread of infectious diseases in a modern world in which humans travel on all scales. We introduce a probabilistic model which accounts for the worldwide spread of infectious diseases on the global aviation network. The analysis indicates that a forecast of the geographical spread of an epidemic is indeed possible, provided that local dynamical parameters of the disease such as the reproduction number are known. The model consists of local stochastic infection dynamics and stochastic transport of individuals on the world-wide aviation network which takes into account the national and international civil aviation traffic. In broad terms, our simulations of the SARS outbreak are in good agreement with published case reports. We propose that our model can be employed to predict the worldwide spread of future infectious diseases and to identify endangered regions in advance. Based on the connectivity of the aviation network we evaluate the performance of different control strategies and show that a quick and focused reaction is essential to inhibit the global spread of epidemics.

11.2 Local infection dynamics

Mathematical models for the description of epidemic outbreaks are rather abundant. Depending on their purpose they differ in their degree of detail (Anderson and May 1991). Some models are designed to reproduce the dynamics of a specific disease with as much accuracy as possible, whereas other models are conceived to reveal the central and general mechanisms underlying an epidemic outbreak. Almost all models share the goal of accounting for the time evolution of the number of infected individuals $I(t)$ in a population of size N. One of the most successful models is the SIR-scheme, in which a population of size N is classified into susceptibles (S), infecteds (I), and recovered/removed (R) individuals. The quantities

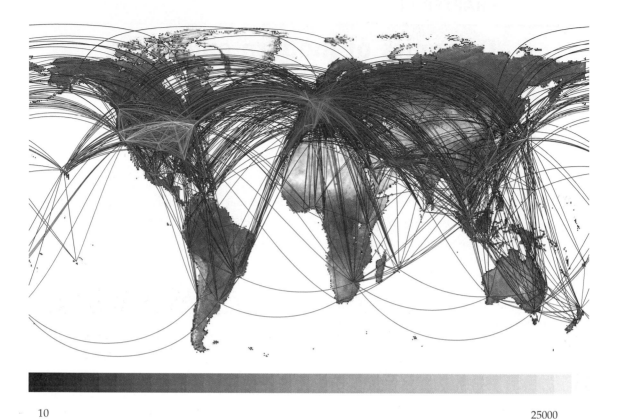

10   25000

Figure 11.1 Global aviation network. A geographical representation of the civil aviation traffic among the 500 largest international airports in over 100 different countries is shown. Each line represents a direct connection between airports. The gray scale of the connections encodes the number of passengers per day (see lower gray code) travelling between two airports. The network accounts for more than 95% of the international civil aviation traffic.

S, I and R are dynamic, while the total number of individuals is conserved, that is,

$$S(t) + I(t) + R(t) = N. \tag{11.1}$$

The infection dynamics are given by

$$\frac{\mathrm{d}S}{\mathrm{d}t} = -\frac{\alpha}{N}SI, \qquad \frac{\mathrm{d}I}{\mathrm{d}t} = \frac{\alpha}{N}SI - \beta I, \tag{11.2}$$

in which it is assumed that the rate of change of susceptibles and infected is proportional to the transmission rate α as well as the concentration of infecteds and susceptibles, respectively. The second term in the second equation takes into account that infecteds recover or are effectively removed from the population at a rate β. The time course of recovereds $R(t)$ is given by the conservation law (11.1). The initial conditions $I(t_0)$ and $S(t_0)$ along with the parameters N, α, and β determine the evolution of the system. The parameter $R_0 = \alpha/\beta$ is known as the reproduction number of the epidemic, that is, the average number of infections transmitted by an infected individual during the period $\tau = \beta^{-1}$ which is the time an infected individual is infectious. A requirement for an epidemic to occur ($\mathrm{d}I/\mathrm{d}t(t_0) > 0$) is a reproduction number greater than unity and an initial relative number of susceptibles $S(t_0)/N > R_0^{-1}$ (assuming that $R(t_0) = 0$). The peak number of infected individuals $I_{\max}$ is given by $I_{\max}/N = 1 - (1 + \ln R_0)/R_0 < 1$. Dividing by the size of the population N and rescaling time as $t \to \beta t$ the dynamics (11.2) can be expressed in terms of the relative concentrations $s = S/N$ and $j = I/N$ of

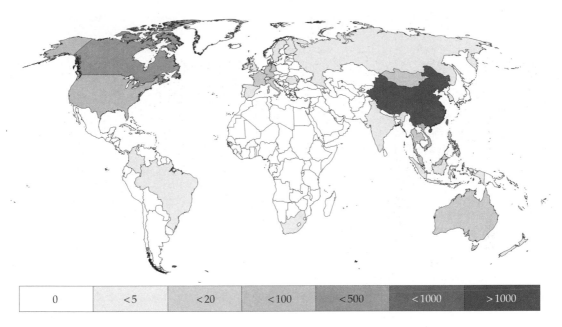

Figure 11.2 Geographical representation of the global spread of probable SARS cases on 30 May 2003 as reported by the World Health Organization (WHO) and the Centers for Disease Control and Prevention (CDC) (Centers for Desease Control and Prevention 2003). The first cases of SARS emerged approximately 5 months earlier in mid November 2002 in Guangdong Province, China.

susceptibles and infecteds respectively and the reproduction number R_0,

$$\frac{\mathrm{d}S}{\mathrm{d}t} = -R_0 sj, \qquad \frac{\mathrm{d}j}{\mathrm{d}t} = R_0 sj - j. \qquad (11.3)$$

Time in Eqn (11.3) is measured in units of the time β^{-1} an individual remains infected. The sole parameter which remains is the reproduction number R_0, the population size has dropped out. This implies for instance that the dynamics of a population with $N = 100,000$ and an initial number of infected $I(t_0) = 100$ exhibits the same dynamics of $j(t)$ as a population with $N = 10,000$ and $I(t_0) = 10$. However, while in population of $N = 100,000$ an initial number of infected $I(t_0) = 5$ makes sense, the analogous initial number of infecteds $I(t_0) = 0.5$ in the population with $N = 10,000$ makes no sense, since there is no such thing as half an infected person. The quantization of individuals is not accounted for by the model defined by Eqn (11.3). In short, ignoring stochastic effects in finite populations, as we have done above, can be a crucial drawback. We will see in the next section that quantization effects are important for they imply a strong impact of the fluctuations of the system which are neglected by the simple deterministic model above.

11.3 The impact of chance

The above SIR model has been able to account for experimental data in a number of cases indicating that Eqn (11.3) incorporate the underlying mechanism of transmission and recovery dynamics. However, transmission of and recovery from an infection are intrinsically stochastic processes and the deterministic SIR model does not account for chance fluctuations. These fluctuations are particularly important at the beginning of an epidemic when the number of infecteds is very small. The understanding of this initial phase of an epidemic is crucial for making any kind of prediction concerning the probability of outbreak in a population and the typical time lag for a given rate of immigration of infecteds.

In order to describe the initial phase, one needs to cast the dynamics of transmission and recovery into a probabilistic model. We begin with the reaction scheme given by

$$S + I \xrightarrow{\alpha} 2I, \quad I \xrightarrow{\beta} \emptyset. \tag{11.4}$$

The first reaction reflects the fact that an encounter of an infected individual with a susceptible results in two infecteds at a probability rate α, the second indicates that infecteds are removed (recover) at a rate β and effectively disappear from the population. The quantity of interest is the probability $p(S, I; t)$ of finding a number S of susceptibles and I infecteds in a population of size N at time t. Assuming that the process is Markovian on the relevant timescales, the dynamics of this probability are governed by the master equation

$$\partial_t p(S, I; t) = \frac{\alpha}{N}(S + 1)(I - 1)p(S + 1, I - 1; t)$$
$$+ \beta(I + 1)p(S, I + 1; t)$$
$$- \left(\frac{\alpha}{N} SI - \beta I\right)p(S, I; t). \tag{11.5}$$

The first term corresponds to the stochastic event $(S + 1, I - 1) \rightarrow (S, I)$, that is a susceptible is infected, the second term to the event $(S, I + 1) \rightarrow (S, I)$, that is an infected recovers from the disease, the third term to the events $(S, I) \rightarrow (S - 1, I + 1)$ and $(S, I) \rightarrow (S, I - 1)$.

The relation of the probabilistic master Eqn (11.5) to the deterministic SIR-model (11.3) is not obvious as the set of equations (11.3) describe the evolution of the quantities $s(t)$ and $j(t)$ whereas the master equation (11.5) describes the evolution of the probability of finding $S(t)$ susceptibles and $I(t)$ infecteds at time t.

However, this gap can be bridged by investigating the master equation in the limit of a large but finite population, that is, $N \gg 1$. In this limit one can approximate the master equation by a Fokker–Planck equation by means of an expansion in terms of conditional moments (Kramers-Moyal expansion, Gardiner 1985) which is a standard technique in the theory of stochastic processes. This procedure yields the associated description in terms of stochastic Langevin equations

$$ds = -R_0 sj\, dt + \frac{1}{\sqrt{N}} \sqrt{R_0 sj}\, dW_1(t) \tag{11.6}$$

$$dj = R_0 sj\, dt - j\, dt - \frac{1}{\sqrt{N}} \sqrt{R_0 sj}\, dW_1(t)$$
$$+ \frac{1}{\sqrt{N}} \sqrt{j}\, dW_2(t) \tag{11.7}$$

having rescaled time as $t \rightarrow \beta t$. Here, the independent Gaussian white noise forces $dW_1(t)$ and $dW_2(t)$ (with $\langle dW_i(t) \rangle = 0$ and $\langle dW_i(t)^2 \rangle = dt$) reflect the fluctuations of transmission and recovery, respectively. Note that the magnitude of the fluctuations are $\propto 1/\sqrt{N}$ and disappear in the limit $N \rightarrow \infty$. In this limit the dynamics (11.6) and (11.7) reduce to the deterministic SIR-model as defined by (11.3) above. However, for large but finite N a crucial difference to Eqn (11.3) is apparent: (1) eqns (11.6) and (11.7) contain fluctuating forces, (2) the population size is a parameter of the system.

For very large, but finite N one expects from Eqns (11.6) and (11.7) that the impact of the noise is small. However, a careful analysis shows that even in this regime, the noise plays a prominent role in the initial phase of an epidemic outbreak and cannot be neglected. Qualitatively this can be understood as follows: assume that initially nearly the entire population is susceptible, that is, $s \approx 1$ and that the disease has an $R_0 > 1$. According to Eqns (11.6) and (11.7) the expected change of the relative number of infecteds $\langle \Delta j \rangle$ in a short time interval Δt is approximately given by

$$\langle \Delta j \rangle \approx (R_0 - 1)j_0 \Delta t, \tag{11.8}$$

where j_0 is the initial relative concentration of infecteds. The relative typical variability of the change Δj relative to the expected change is given by the standard deviation divided by the mean which is of the order of $1/N j_0$, that is,

$$\frac{\sqrt{\langle (\Delta j)^2 \rangle}}{\langle \Delta j \rangle} \approx \frac{1}{N j_0}. \tag{11.9}$$

For arbitrary initial values of j_0 this quotient is a small number. However, in epidemics during the initial phase j_0 is of the order of $1/N$ which implies a variability of order unity. It is important to note that $j = 0$ is an absorbing boundary of the system because if at some point no infecteds are present no epidemic outbreak can occur. Consequently, whether or not an outbreak occurs is a matter of chance. Since any arbitrarily small initial condition $j_0 > 0$ in the deterministic SIR model implies an exponential increase of $j(t)$, it is clear that Eqns (11.3) are of no use in modelling the typical scenario one is confronted with during the initial phase of an epidemic. In the next section we exemplify this reasoning in a system of two coupled populations.

11.4 Interacting populations

Consider the system of two confined populations which exchange individuals as depicted in Fig. 11.3. In each population the dynamics of an epidemic is governed by the simple reaction scheme (11.4). For simplicity we assume that both populations have the same size, that is, $N_A = N_B = N$. In addition to disease transmission and recovery, individuals may traverse from one population to the other at a transition rate γ. Schematically, the entire dynamics is given by

$$S_A + I_A \xrightarrow{\alpha} 2I_A, \qquad I_A \xrightarrow{\beta} \emptyset,$$
$$S_B + I_B \xrightarrow{\alpha} 2I_B, \qquad I_B \xrightarrow{\beta} \emptyset$$
$$I_A \xrightarrow{\gamma} I_B \quad I_B \xrightarrow{\gamma} I_A, \quad S_A \xrightarrow{\gamma} S_B, \quad S_B \xrightarrow{\gamma} S_A,$$

$$(11.10)$$

where the indices label the two distinct populations. The state of the system is given by the probability $p(S_1, I_1, S_2, I_2; t)$ of finding a combination of susceptibles and infecteds in both populations. Along the same lines as presented in the previous section one can construct a master equation for this probability, investigate the limit of large N, and obtain a Fokker–Planck equation in the diffusion limit. Now assume that initially a small number of infected I_0 is introduced to population A without any infecteds contained in B. For a sufficiently high number of infecteds in A an epidemic occurs. For $\gamma > 0$ infecteds are introduced to B and a subsequent outbreak may occur in B after a time lag T. Without noise, that is, in the idealized case of $N \to \infty$ and thus the deterministic SIR-model, any arbitrarily small I_0 triggers two successive outbreaks. This is quite

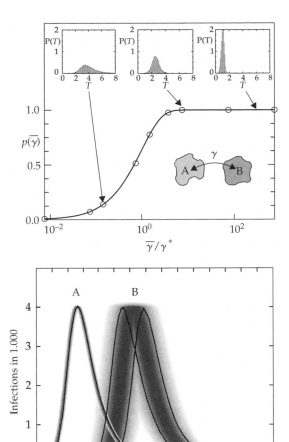

Figure 11.3 Two confined populations with exchange of individuals. In each population the dynamics is governed by the SIR-reaction scheme. Individuals transit from one population to the other at a rate γ. Parameters are $N_A = N_B = 10{,}000$, $R_0 = 4$ and an initial number of infecteds $I_0 = 20$ in population A Left: The probability $p(\gamma)$ of an outbreak occurring in population B as a function of transition rate γ. The insets depict histograms of the time lag T between the outbreaks in A and B for those realization for which an outbreak occurs in B. The circles are results of the simulations of 100,000 realizations, the solid curve is the analytic result of Eqn (11.11) Right: The left black curve represents the time course of $I_A(t)$ of the number if infecteds in population A. The shading reflects the variability of an ensemble of over 100,000 realizations of the process. The trajectories on the right correspond to $I_B(t)$. Two representative realizations are superimposed in black.

different when quantized populations and thus fluctuations are taken into account.

Figure 11.3 depicts the results of simulations for two populations with $N = 10{,}000$ and $R_0 = 4$. Various realizations of the time course $I_A(t)$ and

$I_B(t)$ of the epidemic in both populations were computed. The initial number of infecteds in population A was $I_A(t=0) = I_0 = 20$. The left panel depicts the probability $p(\gamma)$ that the outbreak is followed by an outbreak in population B as a function of the transition rate γ. For large enough rates the probability is nearly unity, since a sufficient number of infecteds is introduced to B. For very low rates γ no infecteds are introduced to B during the time span of the epidemic in A and thus $p(\gamma) \to 0$ as $\gamma \to 0$. For intermediate values of γ the probability $p(\gamma)$ is somewhere in the range $[0,1]$. This means that in this regime one cannot say with certainty whether an epidemic in A is followed by an epidemic in B. This effect is caused by the fluctuations of the system. The function $p(\gamma)$ is given by

$$p(\gamma) = 1 - \exp(-\gamma/\gamma^*), \qquad (11.11)$$

where

$$\gamma^* \approx \left(\frac{R_0 + 1}{R_0 - 1}\right)\frac{1}{2I_{\max}}, \qquad (11.12)$$

is a critical rate which is determined by the parameters N and R_0 of the system and the maximum of infecteds $I_{\max}$ in A. The insets depict histograms of the time lag τ for those realization in which an outbreak occurs in B. Each histogram corresponds to a different transition rate γ. The smaller γ the higher the variability in T. Note that even in a range in which $p(\gamma) \approx 1$ (the right-most of the three insets), the time lag T is still a stochastic quantity with a high degree of variance.

The right panel depicts the infection curves $I_A(t)$ and $I_B(t)$ in both populations. Since $j_A(t=0) \gg 1/N$ in A, the various realizations of $I_A(t)$ nearly coincide. As expected, the impact of fluctuations is small in population A. This is quite different in population B which exhibits a high variability in the time course of $I_B(t)$. Since initially no infecteds are present in this population, the outbreak relies on the immigration of infected from A. Thus, during the initial phase $j_B(t)$ is of the order of $1/N$, the regime in which fluctuations are important. Note, however, that once $j_B(t) \gg 1/N$ the shape of infection curve is relatively uniform and similar to the one predicted by the deterministic model.

Consequently, the introduction of stochastic exchange of infected individuals leads to a lack of predictability in the time of onset of the initially uninfected population. In summary, the investigation of two coupled populations shows that the deterministic SIR-model fails whenever only one population initially contains infected individuals and a full probabilistic description is required.

11.5 Epidemics on networks

The system of two populations can be generalized to an arbitrary number M of populations in a straightforward manner. For simplicity, we assume that the epidemiological parameters α and β and hence the reproduction number R_0 are identical in all populations. In addition to the transmission and recovery dynamics

$$S_i + I_i \xrightarrow{\alpha} 2I_i, \qquad I_i \xrightarrow{\beta} \emptyset, \quad i = 1, \ldots, M, \qquad (11.13)$$

dispersal of individuals is defined by a matrix γ_{ij} of transition rates between populations

$$S_i \xrightarrow{\gamma_{ij}} S_j \qquad I_i \xrightarrow{\gamma_{ij}} I_j, \quad i,j = 1, \ldots, N, \qquad (11.14)$$

where $\gamma_{ii} = 0$. Let us assume that the total number of individuals $\mathcal{N} = \sum_i^M \mathcal{N}_i$ is fixed. For a predefined matrix γ_{ij} the relative concentration of individuals $c_i = N_i/\mathcal{N}$ changes over time. The dynamics of $c_i(t)$ can be interpreted as the probability of finding an individual in population i. This quantity is determined by the master equation for dispersal, that is,

$$\partial_t c_i = \sum_j (\gamma_{ij}c_j - \gamma_{ij}c_i). \qquad (11.15)$$

The stationary state $c_i^* \, i = 1, \ldots, M$ is given by

$$\frac{\gamma_{ij}}{\gamma_{ji}} = \frac{c_i^*}{c_j^*} = \frac{N_i^*}{N_j^*}. \qquad (11.16)$$

In a realistic system, it is reasonable to assume stationarity of dispersal, that is, $N_i(t) \approx N_i^*$ and that the exchange rates between populations fulfill (11.16). Generally, for populations of identical size (i.e. $N_i = N$) the above condition implies that $\gamma_{ij} = \gamma_{ji}$ of every pair (i, j) of populations. Note that this does not imply that all rates are identical, for example, one might have $\gamma_{12} = \gamma_{21}$ and $\gamma_{34} = \gamma_{43}$ but $\gamma_{12} \neq \gamma_{34}$.

Consider a system as depicted in Fig. 11.4. Each population contains N individuals. A central population A is coupled to a set of $M-1$ surrounding populations $B_1, \ldots B_{M-1}$. The exchange rates between the central ($i=0$) and a surrounding population j are the same, that is, $\gamma_{0j} = \gamma_{j0} = \gamma_j$ with $j = 1, \ldots, M-1$. However, the set of rates γ_j can be highly variable.

Assume that initially a number of infecteds I_0 is introduced to the central population A such that an outbreak occurs. Furthermore we assume that there are initially no infecteds in the surrounding populations. The entire set of rates $\{\gamma_j\}_{j=1, \ldots, M-1}$ determines the behaviour in the surrounding populations. If all rates γ_j are identical and very small we expect no infection to occur in the B_j, for large enough γ_j an outbreak will occur in every B_j.

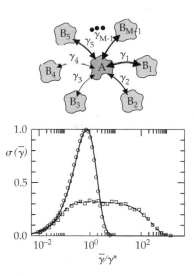

Figure 11.4 Inhomogeneous connections and predictability. Left: A star-like network with a central population A connected to $M-1$ populations $B_1, \ldots, B_M - 1$ with rates $\gamma_1, \ldots, \gamma_M - 1$. Right: The cumulated variance (Eqn 11.9) for a star network with 32 populations is depicted as a function of the average transmission rate $\bar{\gamma}$. Two cases are exemplified: equal rates (circles) and distributed rates according to Eqn (11.19) with $\gamma_{max}/\gamma_{min} \approx 1000$ (squares). The solid and dashed lines shows the analytical results given by Eqns (11.17) and (11.111), respectively. Parameters are N = 10,000 for all populations, $R_0 = 4$ and an initial number of infecteds $I_0 = 20$ in population A. The numerical values are obtained by calculating the variance of the fluctuations of 100 different realizations of the epidemic outbreak for each $\bar{\gamma}$

In a realistic network, however, transition rates are distributed on many scales and the response of the network to a central outbreak depends on the statistical properties of this distribution. We denote the probability density of rates by $\pi(\gamma)$.

In order to quantify the reaction of the network we introduce for each surrounding population a binary number ξ_j with $j = 1, \ldots, M-1$ which is unity if an outbreak occurs in B_j and zero if it does not. The variability of the entire network is quantified be the cumulative variance per population and we define

$$\sigma \equiv \frac{4}{M-1} \sum_i \text{var}(\xi_i)$$
$$= \int d(\gamma)d(\gamma)\,(1-p(\gamma))\pi(\gamma) \qquad (11.17)$$

as a measure for the uncertainty of the network response where $p(\gamma)$ is the probability of outbreak as defined by (11.12). If, for example, all transition rates are identical and equal to $\bar{\gamma}$ (i.e. $\pi(\gamma) = \delta(\gamma - \bar{\gamma})$) one obtains

$$\sigma(\bar{\gamma}) = 4p(\bar{\gamma})(1-p(\gamma)) \qquad (11.18)$$

which is unity for $p(\bar{\gamma}) = \frac{1}{2}$. Comparing with Eqn (11.11) we see that the system with identical transition rates $\gamma_i = \bar{\gamma}$ exhibits the highest degree of unpredictability when the rates are of the order of the critical rate γ^*. The function $\sigma(\bar{\gamma})$ is shown in Fig. 11.4. The assumption of identical transition rates γ_i is never met in real networks of populations. Typically, the transition rates vary considerably between various nodes in a network. Consider for instance the aviation network (Fig. 11.1) where the transport rates vary over many orders of magnitude. The inset depicts a histogram of the flux of individuals from the set of nodes. This indicates that transition rates are distributed on many scales. A high degree of variability in the rates can be accounted for by a probability density

$$\pi(\gamma) = \frac{1}{\log(\gamma_{max}/\gamma_{min})} \frac{1}{\gamma} \quad \gamma_{max} \leq \gamma \leq \gamma_{min}, \qquad (11.19)$$

where the interval $[\gamma_{min}, \gamma_{max}]$ incorporates many orders of magnitude. Inserting into Eqn (11.17) yields $\sigma(\bar{\gamma})$ for strongly distributed rates. In Fig. 11.4 this function is compared to a system of identical transition rates. Clearly, a high variability in rates drastically changes the degree of predictability. On one hand, for intermediate values of $\gamma \approx \gamma^*$ the predictability is much higher than in the system of identical rates. This is a rather counterintuitive result. Despite the additional randomness in transition rates, the degree of determinism is increased. On the other hand, for large values of the average rate $\bar{\gamma}$ predictability is decreased. We conclude that in order to make a reliable prediction on the epidemic spread on a network, one needs an estimate of the distribution of transition rates, that is, the function $\pi(\gamma)$ and its relation to the critical rate γ^* as determined Eqn (11.12).

11.6 The global spread of SARS—a paradigm

The theoretical investigation presented above lead us to investigate the extent to which a worldwide epidemic can be predicted when the local infection parameters such as the reproduction number R_0 as well as the global dispersal parameters are known. A paradigmatic system is the recent worldwide spread of the Severe Acute Respiratory Syndrome (SARS). Figure 11.2 depicts the geographical representation of the global spreading of probable SARS cases on 30 May 2003 as reported by the World Health Organization (WHO) and Centers for Disease Control and Prevention (CDC). The first cases of SARS emerged in mid November 2002 in Guangdong Province, China (Centers for Desease Control and Prevention 2003). The disease was then carried to Hong Kong on 21 February 2003 and began spreading around the world along international air travel routes, as tourists and the medical doctors who treated the early cases travelled internationally. As the disease moved out of southern China, the first hot zones of SARS were Hong Kong, Singapore, Hanoi (Vietnam), and Toronto (Canada), but soon cases in Taiwan, Thailand, the United States, Europe, and elsewhere were reported.

In order to understand the global spread we combined local infection dynamics appropriate for SARS with the stochastic dispersal of individuals on the civil aviation network as depicted in Fig. 11.1.

11.6.1 Local infection dynamics

For the local infection dynamics we chose an extension of the stochastic SIR model similar to Eqn (11.5). The categories S, I, and R are completed by a category L of latent individuals which have been infected but are not infectious yet themselves, accounting for the latency of the disease. In our simulations individuals remain in the latent or infectious stage for periods drawn from a delay distribution (Donnelly *et al.* 2003; Riley *et al.* 2003).

In order to simulate the worldwide spreading of SARS we need to specify the basic reproduction number R_0 and the mean duration of the infectious period $\tau = \beta^{-1}$ of the infection dynamics. For SARS, the distribution of infectious times has been investigated in detail using the case data of the outbreak in Hong Kong (Donnelly *et al.* 2003) The basic reproduction number and how it changed over time is also known (Lipsitch *et al.* 2003; Riley *et al.* 2003).

11.6.2 The aviation network

We collected data which incorporates 95% of the entire civil aviation traffic (IATA 2003). The data comprise flights among the 500 largest international airports in over 100 different countries (AOG 2003). The network considered is depicted in Fig. 11.1. For each pair (i, j) of airports, we checked all flights departing from airport j and arriving at airport i. The amount of passengers carried by a specific flight within one week can be estimated by the size of the aircraft (We used manufacturer capacity information on over 150 different aircraft types) multiplied by the number of days the flight operates in one week. The sum of all flights yields the passengers M_{ij} per week between i and j. The matrix M_{ij} defines the dispersal of individuals on the aviation network. As indicated by the grey code in Fig. 11.1 the matrix elements vary on a number of scales. We computed the total passenger capacity $T_j = \sum_i M_{ij}$ of each airport j per week assuming that flights carry 80% of their capacity and found very good agreement with independently obtained airport capacities.

11.6.3 Modeling dispersal

If we assume that the passenger capacity T_j reflects the need of a catchment area j, this quantity is proportional to the population size N_j at j,

$$N_j \propto T_j. \tag{11.20}$$

Under this assumption the probability w_{ij} that a travelling individual at j is making a transition to i is given by

$$w_{ij} \propto \frac{M_{ij}}{\Sigma_k M_{kj}}. \tag{11.21}$$

Stochastic dispersal of individuals is then governed by the master equation

$$\partial_t P_i = \gamma \sum_j w_{ij} P_j - \gamma P_i, \tag{11.22}$$

where γ is a universal dispersal rate constant which sets the timescale of travelling. The parameter γ can be determined experimentally by measuring the flux of individuals between two arbitrary airports of the network knowing the population sizes of the corresponding catchment areas. The first term in the master equation accounts for the influx of individuals to location i from all other locations j, the second reflects the outflux of individuals from i. In (11.22) the quantity P_i represents any labelled set of individuals. Under the assumption that infecteds I_i and susceptibles S_i exhibit identical dispersal properties, Eqn (11.22) holds for both. We estimated the rate γ by computing the ratio of the number of infected individuals in Hong Kong to the number of infected individuals outside Hong Kong, which is provided by the WHO data.

11.6.4 Results

Figure 11.5(a) depicts a geographical representation of the results of our simulations. Initially, an infected individual was placed in Hong Kong. The basic reproduction number was set to $R_0 = 4.0$ for the first 35 days and subsequently to zero. In a second simulation we chose a time course for $R_0 = 4.0$ for a period of 0–35 days, $R_0 = 1.0$ for days 35–55 and $R_0 = 0.0$ for days 55–∞. Both

simulations lead to similar results. The figure shows the prediction of our model for the spread of SARS 90 days after the initial infection, corresponding to the end of May. We find the results of our simulations to be in remarkable agreement with the worldwide spreading of SARS as reported by the WHO (compare Fig. 11.2): There is an almost one-to-one correspondence between infected countries as predicted by the simulations and the WHO data. Also the numbers of infected individuals in a country agree nicely. This agreement with the reported case seems rather surprising considering that the simulations reflect stochastic single realizations of a stochastic process on a highly coupled network. However, as we have shown in the simple and idealized case investigated in Section 11.5 the high degree of heterogeneity may well increase the predictability and degree of determinism in the system. This is the underlying reason why a forecast of the global spread of an epidemic on the aviation network is indeed feasible.

Figures 11.5(b) and (c) exemplify how our model can be employed to predict endangered regions if the origin of a future epidemic is located quickly. The figures depict simulations of the global spread of SARS 90 days after hypothetical outbreaks in New York and London, respectively. Despite the worldwide spread of the epidemic in each case, the degree of infection of each country differs considerably, which has important consequences for control strategies.

11.7 Control strategies

Vaccination of a fraction of the population reduces the fraction of susceptibles and thus yields a smaller effective reproduction number R_0. If a sufficiently large fraction of the population is vaccinated, R_0 drops below 1 and the epidemic becomes extinct. The global aviation network can be employed to estimate the fraction of the global population that needs to be vaccinated in order to prevent the epidemic from spreading. Figure 11.6 demonstrates that a quick response to an initial outbreak is necessary if global vaccination is to be avoided. The figure depicts the probability $p_n(v)$ of having to vaccinate a fraction v

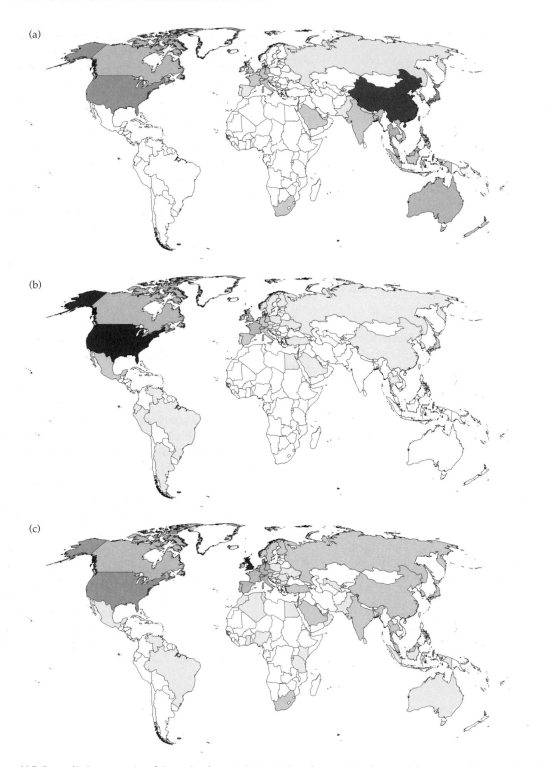

Figure 11.5 Geographical representation of the results of our simulations 90 days after an initial infection in (A) Hong Kong, (B) New York, and (C) London. The same gray code was used as in Fig. 11.2. The simulation in A corresponds to the real SARS infection at the end of May and should be compared to the WHO data shown in Fig. 11.2. Here the worldwide spreading is based on an outbreak starting in Hong Kong in mid February 2003.

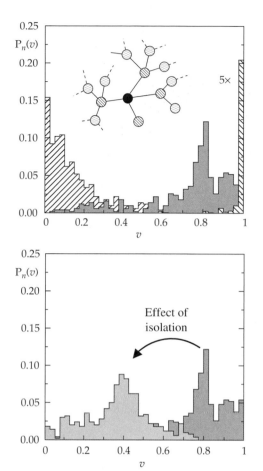

Figure 11.6 Impact and control of epidemics. Left: The probability $p_n(v)$ of having to vaccinate a fraction v of the population in order to prevent the epidemic from spreading, if an initial infected individual is permitted to travel $n=1$ (///), 2 (gray), and 3 (\\\\) times. The probability $p_n(v)$ is estimated by placing the infected individual on a node i (black dot) of the network. The fraction v_n associated with node i is given by the number of susceptibles in the subnetwork defined by the nodes which can be reached by the infected individual after $n=1$, 2, and 3 steps. Histogramming v_i for all nodes i yields an estimate for $p_n(v)$. Right: The quantity $p_2(v)$ exhibits a strong shift to lower values of v when only 2% of the largest cities are isolated after an initial outbreak (light grey) as compared to $p_2(v)$ when no isolation occurs (dark grey).

of the population if an infected individual is randomly placed in one of the cities and permitted to travel $n=1$, 2 or 3 times. For the majority of originating cities the initial spread is regionally confined and thus a quick response to an outbreak requires only a vaccination of a small fraction of the population. However, if the infected individual travels twice, the expected fraction $\langle v \rangle$ of the population which needs to be vaccinated is considerable (74.58%). For $n=3$ global vaccination is necessary.

As a reaction to a new epidemic outbreak, it might be advantageous to impose travel restrictions to inhibit the spread. Here we compare two strategies: (1) the shutdown of individual connections and (2) the isolations of cities. Our simulations show that an isolation of only 2% of the largest cities already drastically reduces $\langle v \rangle$ (with $n=2$) from 74.58% to 37.50% (compare the light-gray and dark grey curves in Figure 11.6). In contrast, a shutdown of the strongest connections in the network is not nearly as effective. In order to obtain a similar reduction of $\langle v \rangle$ the top 27.5% of connections would need to be taken off the network. Thus, our analysis shows that a remarkable success is guaranteed if the largest cities are isolated as a response to an outbreak.

In a globalized world with millions of passengers travelling around the world week by week infectious diseases may spread rapidly around the world. We believe that a detailed analysis of the aviation network represents a cornerstone for the development of efficient quarantine strategies to prevent diseases from spreading. As our model is based on a microscopic description of travelling individuals our approach may be considered a reference point for the development and simulation of control strategies for future epidemics.

CHAPTER 12

The International response to the outbreak of SARS, 2003

David L. Heymann

12.1 Summary

The sudden occurrence of an internationally spreading outbreak of a new and emerging infectious disease in early 2003, severe acute respiratory syndrome (SARS), provided an opportunity for a coordinated international response based on information and evidence obtained in real time through standard and electronic communications. Its containment represents a new way of working internationally, and demonstrates how intense collaboration in virology, clinical medicine, and epidemiology can rapidly provide the information necessary to make and implement evidence-based control measures. The SARS outbreak serves as a reminder of the need for strong national surveillance and response to infectious diseases, evidence-based international travel recommendations, and a global alert, and response network to serve as a safety net when national surveillance fails.

12.2 Regulating the international spread of infectious diseases

The international response to the outbreak of SARS, as it spread from continent to continent during 2003, was in practice the roll out of a proposed, new way of working under the International Health Regulations (IHR) (WHO 1969). The IHR are the only set of international legal rules binding World Health Organization (WHO) member states concerning the control of infectious diseases with potential to spread internationally. The IHR, adopted in 1969, represent a passive system for reporting of three communicable diseases thought to be important because of their potential spread internationally—cholera, plague, and yellow fever. Once reported to WHO, notification is made in *the WHO Weekly Epidemiological Record* describing the geographic extent of the infected area(s). At the same time the IHR describe standard, maximally acceptable measures that may be applied by countries to prevent these diseases from spreading internationally, and sets out norms and standards for sea and airports to prevent the spread of infectious disease vectors from public conveyances that land at these ports.

12.3 Strengthening global alert, global outbreak response, and communication

During the last decade of the twentieth century after several infectious disease outbreaks, including cholera in Latin America, pneumonic plague in India, and Ebola haemorrhagic fever in the Democratic Republic of the Congo, a need was identified for stronger international coordination of outbreak responses, and more timely and accurate information during the course of an outbreak that threatens global public health security. (Anon 1994; Tauxe *et al.* 1995; Heymann 1999; Khan 1999). This led, in 1996, to the start of a revision process of the IHR in order to broaden disease coverage, incorporate the use of more up-to-date communication technologies, and use these up-to-date technologies to provide real-time information on which to formulate measures to prevent international spread (WHO 2002*a*, 2003*h*).

The revision process itself began with a series of field tests that led to the proactive collection of information about disease outbreaks and the development of protocols for coordinated international response, embodied in the Global Outbreak Alert and Response Network (GOARN). GOARN is a network with a secretariat within WHO, that links individual surveillance and response networks that have been established throughout the world. Set up in 1997 and formalized in 2000, it now has over 120 surveillance and response partners worldwide (WHO 1997, 2000; Heymann and Rodier 2001). Though GOARN identifies and responds to more than 50 outbreaks in developing countries each year, the SARS outbreak was the first time that GOARN identified and responded to an outbreak that was rapidly spreading internationally.

One of the partners in GOARN is the WHO Global Influenza Surveillance Network that identifies and tracks antigenic drift and shifts of influenza viruses in order to guide the annual composition of vaccines, and that provides an early alert to variants that might signal the start of a pandemic (WHO 2002b). This network was placed on alert in late November 2002 when the Canadian Global Public Health Intelligence Network (GPHIN), also a partner in GOARN, picked up media reports of an influenza outbreak in mainland China (Health Canada 2002). At the same time another GOARN partner, the US Global Emerging Infections Surveillance and Response System (GEIS), picked up similar media reports about a severe outbreak in Beijing and Guangzhou, with influenza B as the suspected cause. As GOARN continued to receive media and other reports about influenza outbreaks in China, requests for information to Chinese authorities were made by WHO. On 12 December WHO received a detailed report on data collected at Chinese influenza surveillance sites indicating that investigation of 23 influenza virus isolates had confirmed type B strains in all but one, and that the number of cases were consistent with the seasonal pattern in previous years.

Although information is incomplete, retrospective case identification by Chinese and GOARN epidemiologists since May 2003 suggests that there were actually two respiratory disease outbreaks occurring simultaneously in Guangdong Province in late November 2002: influenza, and what now appears to have been the first cases of SARS—an atypical pneumonia that was characterized by small, seemingly unrelated clusters of cases scattered over several municipalities in Guangdong, with low level transmission to healthcare workers (WHO 2003i). This first outbreak of atypical pneumonia appears to have continued until a second outbreak, with amplified transmission to health workers, began during the first 10 days of February. On 10 February 2003, the WHO office in Beijing received an e-mail message describing an infectious disease in Guangdong Province, said to have caused more than 100 deaths. On 11 February the Guangzhou Bureau of Health reported to the press more than 100 cases of an infectious atypical pneumonia outbreak that had been going on in the city for more than a month. That same day the Chinese Ministry of Health officially reported to WHO 300 cases and 5 deaths in an outbreak of acute respiratory syndrome, and the following day reported that the outbreak dated back to 16 November 2002, that influenza virus had not yet been isolated, and that the outbreak was coming under control (Zhong et al. 2003).

When the reports of a severe respiratory disease were received by WHO on 11 February 2003, a new strain of influenza virus was the most feared potential cause and the WHO Global Influenza Network was again alerted. Concern increased on 20 February, when the Network received reports from Hong Kong authorities confirming the detection of A(H5N1) avian influenza virus in two persons, and WHO activated its influenza pandemic preparedness plans (Anon. 2003a,b).

During that same week, laboratories of the WHO Global Influenza Surveillance Network began analysing specimens from a patient with severe atypical pneumonia hospitalized in Hanoi following travel to mainland China and Hong Kong. Concurrently, GOARN response teams in Vietnam and Hong Kong began collecting clinical and epidemiological information about the patient and a growing number of others with similar symptoms.

12.4 Using real-time information for evidence-based control

By 11 March, WHO had enough clinical and epidemiological information to alert the world to the occurrence of a newly identified atypical pneumonia occurring in Asia (WHO 2003*j*). After this alert, reports of more than 150 new cases of atypical pneumonia of unidentified cause were received from hospitals in six Asian countries and Canada (Anon 2003*c*). The disease did not respond to antibiotics and antivirals known to be effective against primary atypical pneumonia and other respiratory infections. No patients, including young and previously healthy health workers, had recovered, many were in critical condition, several required mechanical ventilatory support, and four had died. Equally alarming, the disease was rapidly spreading along the routes of international air travel (see Chapter 11, this volume). The potential for further international spread was clearly demonstrated that same day when a medical doctor, who had treated the first case of atypical pneumonia in Singapore, reported similar symptoms shortly before boarding a flight from New York to Singapore on 14 March. The airline was alerted and the doctor and his wife disembarked in Frankfurt for immediate hospitalization, becoming the first cases in Europe (WHO 2003*k*). On 15 March, WHO therefore issued a second and stronger global alert, this time in the form of an emergency travel advisory (WHO 2003*l*). The alert provided guidance for travellers, airlines and crew, provided a case definition, and gave the new disease its name: SARS. It also launched a coordinated global outbreak response aimed at preventing this newly identified transmissible disease, of undetermined cause and unknown epidemic potential, from becoming endemic.

During the period of outbreak containment GOARN linked some of the world's best laboratory scientists, clinicians, and epidemiologists electronically, in virtual networks that provided rapid knowledge about the causative agent, mode of transmission, and other epidemiological features (WHOMCN 2003). This real-time information made it possible for WHO to provide specific guidance to health workers on clinical management and protective measures to prevent further nosocomial spread. It also made possible a series of recommendations to international travellers to stop its international spread (WHO 2003*k*). Recommendations were at first non-specific, urging international travellers to have a high level of suspicion if they had travelled to or from areas where the outbreak was occurring. But as more information became available that persons with SARS continued to travel internationally by air and were infecting a then unknown number of fellow passengers and that persons were returning home from known SARS-infected areas and becoming ill after their return, airports were asked to screen passengers for history of contact with SARS and for persons with current illness that fit the probable SARS case definition. Finally, when these recommendations did not completely stop international spread, passengers themselves were asked to avoid travel to areas where contact tracing was unable to link all cases to known chains of transmission.

Within 4 months all known chains of transmission of SARS had been interrupted and on 5 July 2003, 20 days after the isolation of the last known probable case, the SARS outbreak was declared contained (WHO 2003*g*). Probable cases of SARS were reported from 27 countries on all continents and through a coordinated effort its international spread had been contained.

12.5 Lessons learned during and after the SARS outbreak

SARS has clearly shown how inadequate surveillance and response capacity in a single country can endanger the public health security of national populations and in the rest of the world. It has also shown how, in a closely interconnected and interdependent world, a new and poorly understood disease, with no vaccine and no effective cure, can adversely affect economic growth, trade, tourism, business and industrial performance, political careers, and social stability. SARS provoked perceptions of personal risk that caused people to wear surgical masks as they went about their daily lives, often in low-risk situations, and provided dramatic images of empty airports and cancelled flights. The perceived risk of SARS was many times greater than the actual risk, a factor that compounded its negative social and economic impact.

SARS has also demonstrated some of the positive features of a globalized society: the advantages that rapid electronic communications and new information technologies bring in responding to emergencies, and the willingness of the international community to form a united front against a shared threat.

Finally, there was an element of good luck that led to the success of the global effort to contain the SARS outbreak: SARS transmitted by droplets during close person-to-person contact and was not transmitted with the same facility as influenza and other infections that are airborne; and SARS did not spread to developing countries where surveillance systems were not sensitive enough to detect its presence before it had spread to others or to potential animal reservoirs. Continued national surveillance for SARS has identified four laboratory workers who appear to have been infected in laboratories handling the virus that caused the outbreak, one worker in Singapore, one in Taiwan, and two in Beijing, and China's national surveillance has identified three laboratory confirmed and one probable case of SARS, all of whom have had a less severe clinical disease (WHO 2003*n,o,p*). Two of these are described in Chapter 5 this volume. With continued national surveillance, and with hypothesis generating for and hypotheses testing of the risk factors of transmission of the SARS Co-Virus from nature to humans, the answers to the many scientific questions generated by the SARS outbreak will eventually be understood. Continued strengthening of GOARN will provide the safety net that will detect and respond to the next emerging disease event of international public health importance should national surveillance again fail to raise the alarm, be it a new and unrecognized agent or the next global pandemic of influenza.

CHAPTER 13

The Experience of the 2003 SARS outbreak as a traumatic stress among frontline health-care workers in Toronto: lessons learned

Robert Maunder, William J. Lancee, Sean B. Rourke, Jonathan Hunter, David S. Goldbloom, Ken Balderson, Patricia M. Petryshen, Molyn Leszcz, Rosalie Steinberg, Donald Wasylenki, David Koh, and Calvin S. L. Fones

13.1 Summary

The outbreak of severe acute respiratory syndrome (SARS) in the first half of 2003 in Canada was unprecedented in several respects. Understanding the psychological impact of the outbreak on healthcare workers, especially those in hospitals is important in planning for future outbreaks of emerging infectious diseases. This review draws upon qualitative and quantitative studies of the SARS outbreak in Toronto to outline factors that contributed to healthcare workers experiencing the outbreak as a psychological trauma. Overall, it is estimated that a high degree of distress was experienced by 29–35% of hospital workers. Three categories of contributory factors were identified. Relevant contextual factors were being a nurse, having contact with SARS patients, and having children. Contributing attitudinal factors and processes were experiencing job stress, perceiving stigmatization, coping by avoiding crowds and colleagues, and feeling scrutinized. Pre-existing trait factors also contributed to vulnerability. Lessons learned from the outbreak include; (1) that effort is required to mitigate the psychological impact of infection control procedures, especially the interpersonal isolation that these procedures promote, (2) that effective risk communication is a priority early in an outbreak, (3) that healthcare workers may have a role in influencing patterns of media coverage that increase or decrease morale, (4) that healthcare workers benefit from resources that facilitate reflection on the effects of extraordinary stressors, and (5) that healthcare workers benefit from practical interventions that demonstrate tangible support from institutions.

13.2 Introduction

The outbreak of SARS following the first known cases in the Guangdong province of China in November, 2002, was extraordinary in the rapidity of its worldwide spread, and the equally impressive rapidity of the identification and characterization of the coronavirus that caused the infection. The outbreak was also unusual for the high rate of infection among hospital workers. The infectiousness of SARS was substantially higher in hospital settings prior to accurate identification of the syndrome and institution of isolation precautions (mean number of secondary cases transmitted from each case, $R_0 = 4$) (WHO 2003f) than it was in hospitals after isolation precautions were in place ($R_0 < 1$) (Low and McGeer 2003) or in the community ($R_0 < 1$) (Low 2004).

Unfortunately, there was little precedent in the medical literature by which to anticipate the psychological effects of the infection within SARS-affected hospitals. Efforts to deal with the psychological stress of healthcare workers were guided instead by general principals of stress response and adaptation, availability of local resources, and responsiveness to emerging patterns of psychological resilience and vulnerability.

Although the psychological stress that has been caused by large-scale events such as natural disasters (Steinglass and Gerrity 1990; Johnsen et al. 1997) and hostile acts (Galea et al. 2003) has been described, there were features of the SARS outbreak that made it unlike other stressors. Because so little is known about the psychological impact of large-scale infectious threats within hospitals, and the psychological impact of the measures that are required to contain infection, it is the purpose of this chapter to review the observations that have been made of the psychological impact of SARS on healthcare workers in order to draw lessons from this experience that may be valuable in the support of hospital staff in the future as new infectious diseases emerge.

The primary sources of information used for this review are the observations made early in the outbreak by mental health professionals and administrators at Mount Sinai Hospital (Maunder et al. 2003), and a survey of 1557 healthcare workers at three Toronto hospitals performed in late May and early June 2003 (Lancee et al. 2004). Where possible, these observations are supplemented by the observations of the psychological impact of SARS on healthcare workers made by other researchers (Maunder et al. 2003; McBride 2003; McGillis Hall et al. 2003; Chan and Huak 2004; Robertson et al. 2004) and, where necessary, by the authors' anecdotal observations of clinical work.

13.3 Characteristics of the outbreak in Toronto

In Toronto SARS occurred in two waves. A woman travelled with SARS from Hong Kong to Toronto on 23 February. She died at home but her son (Case A), who cared for her, went to hospital with respiratory symptoms on 7 March. Seven cases became infected through contact with Case A, including four family members, two patients who had contact with him in hospital, and one technologist. By 16 March, contact with these cases had been responsible for 45 further cases, including 30 healthcare workers (Poutanen et al. 2003; Varia et al. 2003). The first wave peaked in late March and the second wave peaked in late May. In all, there were 375 suspected and probable cases of SARS in the province of Ontario, most of those in the city of Toronto, and 44 deaths (Health Canada 2003). Healthcare workers accounted for over 40% of those infected with SARS in Toronto, and three healthcare workers died (National Advisory Committee on SARS and Public Health 2003).

The hospital milieu changed abruptly in late March. A command structure was put in place in hospitals and public health directives from the province were enacted authoritatively. Physical access to each hospital was restricted to a single entrance. Researchers, students, volunteers, and hospital workers whose work was deemed non-essential to patient care were told to stay home. Visitors were not allowed, with some exceptions. Surgical procedures and outpatient appointments were cancelled. Infection control procedures took precedence over almost all other aspects of hospital function.

13.4 Limited state of knowledge early in outbreak

Although we can now be confident that the cause of SARS is a coronavirus (Berger et al. 2004), and that its human-to-human transmissibility is relatively low (Low and McGeer 2003; WHO 2003f), during the time period of March–May 2003 this was not known. The coronavirus as a putative cause of SARS was identified in scientific papers in May (Drosten et al. 2003; Ksiazek et al. 2003; Peiris et al. 2003a). Furthermore, frontline hospital workers represent a wide range of expertise and biological sophistication. Healthcare workers at this stage of the outbreak had to tolerate uncertainty, and to weigh conflicting claims about personal risk from many sources.

Thus, to understand the psychological impact of the SARS outbreak one needs to appreciate the circumstance of dealing with an unknown infectious pathogen, with an unknown mode of transmission, which appears to be highly contagious and frequently fatal, while having as one's main source of defence the rapidly changing recommendations of experts and administrators for which the rationale is not always immediately apparent. Understandably the normative experience was of considerable stress.

13.5 Methodology of the survey of healthcare workers

The survey instrument comprised the Impact of Event Scale (IES) (Horowitz *et al.* 1979) and the Study of Healthcare Workers' Perception of Risk and Preventive Measures for SARS, a self-report questionnaire authored by two of us (C.S.L.F., D.K.). The survey included 76 survey items probing attitudes towards SARS, infection control procedures, perceived risk, and coping. Attitude statements were scored on a 6-point scale from 1 (strongly disagree) to 6 (strongly agree). Because the outbreak was unprecedented, and because the information required was specific to the outbreak, there was no opportunity to validate the SARS survey against other measures of coping and perceived risk. Surveys were not included in the analysis if more than 15 attitudinal items were missing or if any IES item was missing.

The IES is a measure of traumatic stress comprising 15 items probing the frequency of attitudes related to a particular event, specified as the SARS outbreak. Items probe intrusion, for example, 'I had waves of strong feelings about it,' and avoidance, for example, 'I stayed away from reminders of it'. Responses are never (scored 0), rarely (1), sometimes (3), and often (5) regarding the 1-week period preceding the survey (Horowitz *et al.* 2000; Sundin and Horowitz 2003). The validity and reliability of the scale are well documented (Horowitz *et al.* 2000). A total IES score greater than 19 is considered high (Horowitz *et al.* 2000), and this cut-off was adopted to indicate clinical significance in this analysis.

Two items were added to the survey to probe relationship styles which previous research indicates as being relevant to outcomes of health

related stresses (Hunter and Maunder 2001; Maunder and Hunter 2001). These items were selected from the Experience in Close Relationships—revised questionnaire, a self-report measure of attachment insecurity (Fraley *et al.* 2002). In a sample of 22,494 subjects who have completed this instrument on the Internet (data courtesy of Dr C. Fraley, Chicago, IL) the correlation of the item 'I often wish that my partner's feelings for me were as strong as my feelings for him or her' is 0.74 to the full anxious attachment subscale, and is 0.11 to the avoidant attachment subscale. The correlation of the item 'I feel uncomfortable sharing my private thoughts and feelings with my partner' is 0.63 to the full avoidant attachment subscale, and 0.14 to the anxious attachment subscale. For the SARS survey 'my partner' was changed to 'others'.

Between-group differences in total IES score are used to illustrate the effects of various factors that were related to traumatic stress in healthcare workers. To illustrate the relationship between IES score and continuous variables, healthcare workers have been divided into groups with low, moderate, and high scores by a tertile split of all subjects.

To illustrate the additive clinical effect of independent factors acting on IES, continuous variables which were significantly associated with total IES scores in a hierarchical regression analysis (Lancee *et al.* 2004), were recoded as dichotomous variables (agree or strongly agree = 1, any other response = 0). Healthcare workers were then categorized by the number of risk factors present and the prevalence of high IES scores (total score >19) was calculated for each category.

13.6 The impact of the outbreak on hospital workers

Among the 1557 Toronto hospital workers surveyed in May and June of 2003, the mean level of intrusion was 7.73 (95% confidence interval 7.37–8.11) and of avoidance was 9.57 (9.16–9.98), and the mean total IES score (combining both dimensions) was 16.84 (16.14–17.54).

Alternatively, to calculate an overall impression of the magnitude of the impact of a stressor, one can count the number of people who report a stress response above a cut-off. The number of subjects in the survey of 3 Toronto hospitals with a total IES score >19 was 561 or 36.0% of the sample. This rate is quite similar to the rate that was found among hospital workers in Singapore by two of us (C.S.L.F, D.K.). At another large Toronto teaching hospital distress caused by SARS (a score on the 12-item general health questionnaire (GHQ) >3) was found in 29% of hospital workers (Nickell *et al.* 2004). At a general hospital in Singapore, a GHQ score above the case cut-off was found in 27% of hospital workers (Chan and Huak 2004).

13.6.1 Impact on particular groups of healthcare workers

Contact with SARS patients
Having direct clinical responsibility for patients with suspected or probable SARS and persons under investigation for SARS is an obvious source of SARS related stress. Hospital workers who cared for SARS patients had a mean IES score of 20.94 (19.41–22.46) whereas those without such contact had a mean score of 15.45 (14.68–16.21).

Professional discipline
The survey was completed by a broad array of different types of hospital workers, proportionately similar to the make up of the hospitals that we surveyed. Nurses experienced the most severe stress and physicians the least, with other hospital workers reporting a mean IES score that was intermediate (Fig. 13.1). The same pattern of distribution between disciplines was reported at another hospital using the GHQ to measure distress (Nickell *et al.* 2004).

Healthcare workers who are parents
Many healthcare workers noted the difficulty of returning home from work to family, especially when there were children present at home. Although most hospital workers did not believe that their loved ones were at high risk (60.1% disagreed or disagreed strongly with the statement 'I feel that people close to me have been at high risk'), anecdotally, hospital workers reported worry about passing on infection. Other concerns expressed included worries about the stigma that might be experienced by family members

(Robertson *et al.* 2004) and worries about how children would be cared for if the healthcare worker-parent were hospitalized or quarantined.

In spite of the general disagreement that close family members were at high risk, the survey data indicate that having children was associated with significantly higher score on the Impact of Event scale (Fig. 13.2). Having children was also identified as a factor contributing to greater distress as measured by the GHQ-12 (Nickell *et al.* 2004).

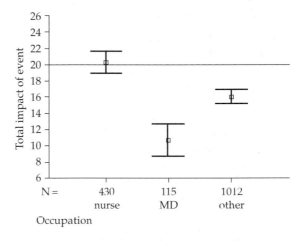

Figure 13.1 Relationship of impact of event score to professional discipline in hospital workers during SARS outbreak. The figure shows mean IES score and the error bars are 95% confidence intervals around the mean.

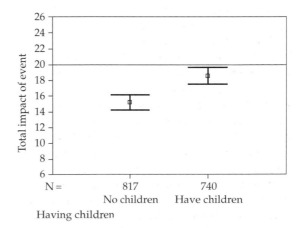

Figure 13.2 Relationship of impact of event score to having children in hospital workers during SARS outbreak. The figure shows mean IES score and the error bars are 95% confidence intervals around the mean.

13.6.2 Mediating factors

Social isolation

One of the ways in which the SARS outbreak was extraordinary among stressful events was the way in which it isolated healthcare workers from their peers, families, and communities. There were many changes during the outbreak that contributed to isolation. Restrictions on access left the hospital considerably emptier than normal. There were also a variety of restrictions on contact. Healthcare workers were instructed to avoid unnecessary contact. Handshaking is an example of a common type of physical contact that was not allowed. Meetings of even a few people within the hospital were discouraged. Staff members were advised not to meet with one another outside of the hospital.

When there was conversation, it occurred through the barriers of protective equipment. The equipment required varied with context and with time, as precautions were altered over the course of the outbreak. The minimum protective equipment intervening between two participants in a dialogue included masks. However, when seeing patients or working in more sensitive areas of the hospital more equipment was required, including perhaps a plastic eye shield or goggles, mask, double gloves, one or two gowns, a hair net, and surgical greens. Identifying oneself became the mandatory starting point of most conversations. Most healthcare workers reported difficulty wearing masks, almost half (47%) because of difficulty communicating while wearing a mask (Nickell *et al.* 2004).

Our survey data show that, although healthcare workers were instructed to avoid colleagues and large meetings, staff who reported coping with concerns about infection by avoiding crowds and colleagues were experiencing a more intense stress response (Fig. 13.3).

Stigma

Another form of social isolation was the disconnection from community experienced by healthcare workers who perceived that people were avoiding contact with them. Many healthcare workers reported others avoiding or cancelling social engagements or avoiding casual contact in

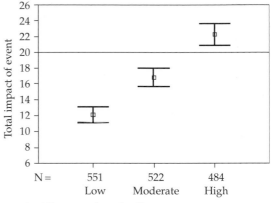

Figure 13.3 The relationship of impact of event score to the response of hospital workers to two attitude statements about avoidance. The statements were: 'I have personally coped with the SARS situation by avoiding crowds and colleagues' and 'I have personally coped with the SARS situation by avoiding crowded places'. Low, moderate, and high categories are determined by a tertile split of mean score on these items. The figure shows mean IES score and the error bars are 95% confidence intervals around the mean.

the community. The SARS outbreak continued through the Easter and Passover celebrations which lead to tensions within the families of many healthcare workers.

Media coverage of healthcare workers may have influenced public perception. In one highly publicized case, a nurse who rode a passenger train before being diagnosed and hospitalized with suspected SARS was vilified in the press. A subsequent qualitative analysis of the image of nurses in the Toronto media revealed that stigmatizing responses were a common theme (McGillis Hall *et al.* 2003).

Healthcare workers who perceived that they or their families were being avoided by others were experiencing a more intense stress response (Fig. 13.4). Similarly, healthcare workers who felt that they were being treated differently by people because of working in a hospital were more likely to have a higher concern for their personal health (Nickell *et al.* 2004).

Scrutiny

Another factor that may have contributed to stress was the unusual degree of scrutiny received by hospital workers from various sources. A high

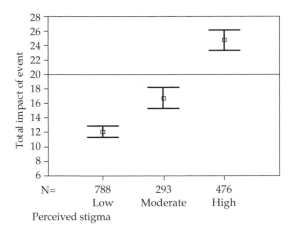

Figure 13.4 Relationship of impact of event score to perceived stigma in hospital workers during SARS outbreak. The figure shows mean IES score and the error bars are 95% confidence intervals around the mean.

level of vigilance of the daily health of all health-care workers by the hospital was evident in, for example, the screening process through which each staff member passed at the start of each shift. A list of questions regarding recent symptoms and recent contacts was asked by screening personnel at the door and then the staff member's temperature was taken. Symptoms probed included non-specific symptoms such as headache and feeling unwell. This process, although very useful for case detection, may also have contributed to anxious hyper-vigilance of one's own symptoms for the rest of the day. It was not unusual for healthcare workers to measure their own temperatures, for example, several times a day. In the survey 349 of 1557 healthcare workers (22.4%) indicated that they agree or strongly agree with the statement 'I have been preoccupied with my own physical symptoms'. Another source of scrutiny was the coverage of the outbreak and the response of hospitals in the media.

Job stress
The SARS outbreak may have influenced stressful job conditions in a number of ways. Being assigned to unfamiliar tasks was stressful for some healthcare workers, such as non-clinical staff who were reassigned to screening duties or other unfamiliar tasks. Seventy-one of the 102 healthcare

workers (70%) who had been working as door screeners indicated they agreed or strongly agreed that 'I have felt more stressed at work'. The correlation co-efficient between the response to the survey items 'I have had to do work that I don't normally do' and 'I have felt more stressed at work' was 0.38 ($p < 0.001$).

Conflict between co-workers was also made more likely by the circumstances. Substantial differences in the status of various healthcare workers during the outbreak (e.g. those designated 'non-essential' or not, those required to work on a SARS isolation unit or not) ensured that there would be comparisons made between one person's lot and another's. In addition, administrative decisions were required as to whether healthcare workers would be given a choice about working in SARS treatment areas and whether staff directly caring for SARS patients would receive pay premiums. There was no mechanism in place to ensure that the same administrative choices would be made at different hospitals.

Changes in workload were also associated with feeling more work stress—particularly increases in workload and overtime. Anecdotally, managers reported difficulty going home at the end of a work day because of a sense of responsibility for their staff. Staff members who usually work part-time at more than one institution were not allowed to do this and as a result were working too little and had financial concerns.

In analysis of the survey data a factor comprising of general feelings of work stress, increased workload, and increased reporting of conflict between co-workers was associated with higher levels of reporting a traumatic stress response to SARS (Fig. 13. 5).

13.6.3 Individual traits that contribute to stress

The survey included a measure of one trait, insecure attachment, which probes the quality of close interpersonal relationships. In particular we measured the degree to which people acknowledged anxious dependence on their partner, and difficulty sharing thoughts and feelings. Previous work suggests that these aspects of relationship style are relatively enduring personal characteristics that may contribute to psychological outcomes of health problems (Maunder and Hunter 2001).

Although the need to keep the survey brief necessitated using only a single item to probe each of those qualities, this measure nonetheless turned out to be a significant predictor of outcome. As opposed to each of the other mediating factors discussed, there were no between-group differences in attachment insecurity when comparing groups based on professional discipline, contact

with SARS patients, and having children, which is what is expected for a trait factor that pre-existed the SARS crisis. In hierarchical regression, after controlling for the effects of each of the group factors and mediating factors described above, attachment insecurity made an independent further contribution to explain variance in total IES (Lancee *et al.* 2004).

13.6.4 Cumulative effect of multiple factors contributing to stress

In regression analysis of survey factors associated with total IES, seven factors were found to be significantly associated with the severity of stress response. These were direct care of probable and suspected SARS patients, being a nurse, having children, experiencing job stress, experiencing social rejection, coping through avoidance of crowds and colleagues, and attachment insecurity (Lancee *et al.* 2004). Figure 13.6 illustrates the cumulative effects of multiple independent risk factors on high-stress outcomes in the SARS outbreak. In this graph the likelihood of a high IES score increased with each additional risk factor present such that for the 681 healthcare workers who had 4 or more risk factors, the risk of a high IES score was greater than 50%. This high risk group represents 43% of the total sample.

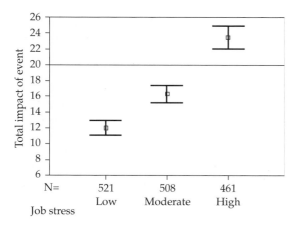

Figure 13.5 Relationship of impact of event score to job stress in hospital workers during SARS outbreak. The figure shows mean IES score and the error bars are 95% confidence intervals around the mean.

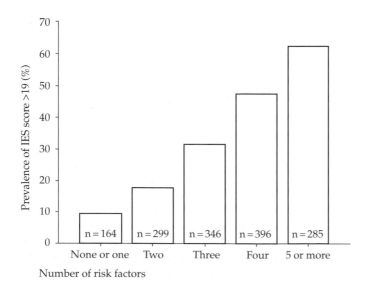

Figure 13.6 Proportion of healthcare workers experiencing SARS outbreak as a psychological trauma by number of risk factors present. Risk factors are: (1) exposure to SARS patients; (2) having a child; (3) being a nurse; (4) perceived social rejection; (5) behavioral avoidance; (6) job stress; and (7) attachment insecurity.

13.7 Discussion

In the public perception, the SARS outbreak turned the modern world of healthcare on its head in Toronto, in the sense that healthcare workers were seen as victims and vectors of disease rather than healers and hospitals were seen as contaminated areas rather than places fostering health. Uncertainty and fear were the intertwined forces that propelled a substantial stress response in many people, particularly healthcare workers.

It deserves emphasis that several of the risk factors for stress, identified anecdotally or through analysis of survey data, have in common the potential to increase one's sense of isolation from peers, family, or community. Social support is known to be one of the most effective buffers against the adverse effects of life-stress (Callaghan and Morrisey 1993; Uchino *et al*. 1996) and so the isolating effects of SARS may have been its most potently provocative feature. These isolation-provoking factors include: first, the experience of social stigma, which separated healthcare workers from members of their community with whom they might otherwise have engaged constructively. Second, choosing to avoid others in crowds or choosing to avoid colleagues appears to have contributed to stress, even though such avoidance was recommended as a public health precaution. Interpersonal contact was diminished by the necessity of using personal protective equipment, especially masks, which greatly reduced the ability to communicate with the nuances of non-verbal expression, and even interfered with healthcare workers recognizing one another. Finally, individuals with a relationship style that makes it more difficult to benefit from available support (Maunder and Hunter 2001) were at even greater risk. Thus, one of the factors that makes SARS unique among recent large-scale stressors was the constellation of factors that each contributed to a sense of isolation among healthcare workers.

The association between professional discipline and SARS stress requires further discussion. Possible explanations are that there were pre-existing discipline-specific differences in levels of stress, or that disciplines are dissimilar in their association to factors that predispose to traumatic stress reactions (such as prior history of psychiatric illness or prior experience with psychological trauma). A third possibility is that this difference relates to differences in the intensity of contact with patients, such as the total duration of time spent with patients, which was not measured in the survey. Finally, disciplines may differ in the degree to which they experience the impact of various mediating factors. For example, if nurses value stress-reducing conversations with their co-workers more than other healthcare workers do, then nurses will be more greatly affected by sanctions against collegial contact.

The mean values of IES scores allow the impact of the SARS outbreak to be compared to the impact of other large-scale stressors that have been assessed using the same instrument and recently reviewed (Sundin and Horowitz 2003). In this comparison, the intensity of stress experienced during the SARS outbreak ranks slightly below that measured 2 weeks (Johnsen *et al*. 1997) to 16 weeks (Steinglass and Gerrity 1990) after a natural disaster. These comparisons require attention to the time elapsed between the stressor and measurement of IES. More time passing before measurement of impact usually results in lower levels of distress. The comparison is further complicated by difficulty in identifying the time between stressor and measurement in SARS because the outbreak was not a discrete event, like a natural disaster, but occurred over many weeks.

The significance of a high rate of high IES scores shortly after the peak of the outbreak also depends on the degree to which high distress is likely to be maintained over a long period of time, and the degree to which distress is associated with impaired function. These questions cannot be answered by the empirical evidence currently available. Previous studies of the chronicity and impact of traumatic stress symptoms suggest that posttraumatic symptoms occurring in the month after exposure to an event often resolve spontaneously rather than persisting as posttraumatic stress disorder. Studies of other traumatic stressors suggest that symptoms of posttraumatic stress disorder occurring immediately after a stressful event resolve in 6% of persons within a few weeks, in 53% of persons after 3 months and in 58% of persons after 9 months (Shalev *et al.* 1998), but clearly, more research into the long-term effects of SARS is required.

13.7.1 Lessons learned

Given the human cost of the SARS outbreak and the potential for much greater adversity with future emerging disease, it is important to learn from our experience. With this in mind, the following lessons draw inferences that go somewhat beyond the data. Where possible these suggestions for future practice follow directly from empirical research, our own and others. When there is no such data available, inferences are drawn from anecdotal observations during SARS and general principles of adaptation and crisis management.

Consider and mitigate the adverse effects of interpersonal isolation
The first of the lessons learned from SARS from a psychological perspective is that the costs of interpersonal isolation need to be borne in mind when widespread infection control procedures are implemented. To the extent that acute traumatic stress interferes with functional abilities within a healthcare setting, this is an issue that relates not only to the comfort of healthcare workers but also to the effectiveness of healthcare in general, at a time when attention to detail and professionalism are of vital importance.

It is not possible to eliminate the isolating effects of an infectious outbreak. Procedures that reduce interpersonal contact are essential to controlling an emerging infectious disease. However, it should be recognized that there may be a substantial cost to the well-being of healthcare workers, at least in the short-run. The impact of social isolation as it relates to visitor policies for hospital patients and people in quarantine was recognized as a significant consequence of SARS in a public review of lessons learned from SARS in Ontario, leading to recommendations for careful case-by-case evaluation of the need for contact restrictions, following clear and sensible rules (Ontario Expert Panel on SARS and Infectious Disease Control 2004). A similar approach to site-by-site evaluation of the degree of contact restrictions required for hospital

personnel may be valuable. However, common sense dictates that there is no psychological benefit in allowing an infectious outbreak to escape control.

Even when the relative interpersonal isolation of healthcare workers is unavoidable, effort should be made to design other measures to increase communication and interpersonal support to mitigate against the inevitable stress of the situation. Ingenuity is required to diminish interpersonal isolation. Various modalities of communication that were exploited during SARS at various settings included enhanced use of e-mail and hospital intranet and internet facilities, telephone messaging, 'buddying' of healthcare workers in higher risk areas, formal and informal telephone and fax networks (especially for quarantined workers), and telephone help-lines (Maunder *et al.* 2003; McBride 2003).

Attend to the popular perception of infectious risk and the costs and benefits of authoritative action
One aspect of the SARS outbreak that is very likely to be shared by future outbreaks was the very limited knowledge available early in the outbreak, which provides a volatile fuel for anxiety. After the experts acquire knowledge, the task of communicating risk information effectively is complex and requires knowledge of the contextual factors that affect appreciation of risk (Alaszewski and Horlick-Jones 2003). In the SARS outbreak, even with the extraordinary transparency and international cooperation that occurred in the scientific community after World Health Organization (WHO) issued a global alert on 12 March 2003, there were nonetheless substantially different levels of awareness of knowledge among expert investigators, clinicians, public officials, and the lay public.

The net result of gradually accumulating knowledge and subsequent difficulties in adequately communicating risk information is a protracted period of uncertainty. During such a period it may be difficult or impossible to achieve public consensus about key issues, such as the necessity for large-scale isolation precautions. When authoritative action is taken to ensure that infection control efforts are concerted and effective, the psychological impact of the infectious event may be affected both by uncertainty and by reactions to the imposition of rules, responsibilities, and limitations. It is an important empirical question to determine the costs and benefits of authoritative leadership.

Attend to the effect of media portrayals of healthcare workers

The apparent impact of media scrutiny and stigma draw attention to the importance of the media as a potential mutative factor in healthcare worker stress. During the SARS outbreak in Toronto inaccurate portrayals of healthcare workers that fostered a stigmatizing view, were prominent in the media (McGillis Hall *et al.* 2003), especially early in the outbreak. A different theme, the description of nurses as heroes (McGillis Hall *et al.* 2003), occurred somewhat later. This shift in media coverage appeared to have an immediate, positive impact on the morale of healthcare workers, and may have been influenced by efforts within the healthcare community to correct misinformation and to provide the media with an alternative narrative. This serves as an example of an opportunity for leaders within the healthcare community to have a positive influence on the well-being of healthcare workers through their contact with the popular media.

Provide time, space, and expertise to foster reflection and adaptation

Effective coping with serious health-related stressors can be fostered by understanding the effects of the stressor as a normal response to an extraordinary event and by focussing attention upon the range of coping activities that are available (problem-solving, emotion-based coping, and meaning-focussed coping) (Folkman and Greer 2000). One of us (ML) met several times after the SARS outbreak with willing ICU staff, employing a group format that focussed explicitly on the issues of normal people dealing with extraordinary events. The usual atmosphere of work in intensive care or in emergency medicine is highly reactive and fast-paced. Providing the time and space for reflection and support requires both staff and the hospital's leadership to recognize the importance of maintaining our own resilience in the face of a crisis.

Provide practical support

Perhaps most obviously, staff members need practical support, such as the reassurance that their livelihood is not at risk if they are not able to work due to illness or infection control precautions. There may be substantial psychological benefit in providing adequate training and adequate supplies of personal protection equipment.

The most effective forms of support are not always obvious. For example, intensive care nurses at one centre united around a demand to be provided with surgical greens for work. The hospital determined that greens were not necessary for infection control. Providing greens is expensive and theft of greens is a frequent problem. Although experts might agree that greens are not necessary to control infectious spread, individual workers were well aware that accepted models of viral transmission had not been 100% accurate throughout the outbreak and that the experts had made mistakes. Some workers reported that they changed their clothes in the garage at night rather than taking the risk that a SARS virus living on the fabric might come in contact with a family member. One approach to remedy this disagreement would be an intensive effort to educate nurses about the limited benefits of greens, but that approach would risk further alienating a vitally important group of healthcare workers. Instead, recognizing that the psychological impact of perceived support and personal control is important, a negotiation took place in which the nurses devised a system of signing out greens to prevent theft, and the hospital ensured an adequate supply. The negotiation was empowering for healthcare workers and boosted morale.

In summary, much has been learned about the acute effect of the SARS outbreak on hospital workers, and some lessons have been drawn that merit testing in the unfortunate but likely event of further outbreaks of unfamiliar infectious diseases. This work, of course, leaves many questions. We do not know whether stress symptoms related to SARS persist in our hospital workers or whether the acute stress has largely returned to normal. We do not know the prevalence of posttraumatic stress disorder related to SARS. We do not know the degree to which SARS has contributed to professional burnout. And perhaps most importantly for the system as a whole, we do not know what the effect of the SARS outbreak has been on the ability of hospitals and professional schools to recruit new staff, to retain the staff that they have, and to train professionals to work in emergency medicine and intensive care. Finally, although healthcare in Toronto was greatly changed for several weeks during the SARS outbreak, we do not yet know the different effects that may have occurred in regions like China where the impact of infection, death, and extensive infection control procedures was much greater.

Throughout the world, hundreds of healthcare workers acquired SARS and some died. It appears likely that thousands more were traumatized, at least acutely, by their SARS experience. The lessons that we learn and apply to future events are critical to the well-being and competent functioning of the healthcare workers who will serve at the frontline in the next battle against an emerging infection.

CHAPTER 14

Informed consent and public health

Onora O'Neill

14.1 Summary

During the last 25 years, medical ethics has concentrated largely on clinical medicine and the treatment of individual patients. This focus permits a view of medical provision as a (quasi) consumer good, whose distribution can be or should be contingent on individual choice. The approach cannot be extended to public health provision. Public health provision, including measures for limiting the spread of infectious diseases, is a public good, and can be provided for some only if provided for many. The provision, or non-provision, of public goods cannot be contingent on individual informed consent, so must be in some respects compulsory. An adequate ethics of public health needs to set aside debates about informed consent and to consider the permissible limits of just compulsion for various types of public good. It will therefore gain more from engaging with work in political philosophy than with individualistic work in ethics.

14.2 Informed consent in medical ethics

Medical ethics has been transformed during the past 30 years. One conspicuous change has been a steadily increasing focus on informed consent, which is now usually taken to be essential for any ethically acceptable medical practice. The literature on informed consent in medical ethics is vast and repetitive. However, it has significant limitations. Some of the difficulties are well known and recalcitrant, although this seldom dents the enthusiasm of those who think informed consent essential to (or even sufficient for) ethically acceptable medical practice. In this chapter, I shall mention the commonly discussed difficulties, but concentrate on some less discussed but philosophically deeper difficulties that limit the use to which informed consent procedures can be put in public health provision.

Some of the most frequent disagreements about informed consent are about the basic reasons for thinking that is ethically important. Is informed consent required in order to respect persons or in order to respect the autonomy of persons? If the latter, which conception of autonomy is relevant? If some persons are more autonomous than others, will informed consent procedures be more important for them? Or will they, on the contrary, be more important for those with limited autonomy? Alternatively, are informed consent procedures required because they provide a degree of assurance that patients are not deceived or coerced in the course of clinical practice? (Faden and Beauchamp 1986; Wolpe 1998; O'Neill 2002*a*)

A second, even more frequently discussed, range of problems arises when patients cannot grasp the information that is essential to giving informed consent. If they cannot understand the proposition to which their consent is sought, they cannot give or refuse informed consent. The hard cases are numerous and intractable. Many patients cannot consent to medical intervention or treatment because they are too young, too ill, too disabled, or too demented to understand the information that they would have to grasp in order to make an informed choice. As they can hardly be denied medical treatment because of these difficulties, it must be given without their consent. Should it then be given on the basis of others' consent (e.g. that of parents, guardians, or relatives)? Or does the very idea of proxy consent undermine the fundamental concerns that are taken to justify informed consent requirements, or even show disrespect for individuals or their autonomy? Should proxy consent perhaps be set aside as mere pretence, and replaced with greater reliance on professional judgement of each patient's best interests? Or would doing so revert to unacceptable medical paternalism, so fail to respect patients and their (faltering) autonomy? Responses to these questions often propose ways of revising or refining the procedures used for requesting and recording consent in order to make consenting easier for less competent patients. But even the most energetic and time consuming presentation of user-friendly information, even the most elaborate and detailed consent forms and procedures, will not make informed consent possible for numerous patients with various types of incapacity.

However, these are not the deepest difficulties. Informed consent procedures are problematic not merely because their philosophical rationale is disputed, and not merely because some individuals lack competence to consent, or lack it at some times. The most basic philosophical difficulties with informed consent arise because consent is a propositional attitude. Consenting—like other cognitive states or acts such as knowing, believing, understanding, hoping, wondering, thinking, desiring, or fearing—takes a proposition as its object. Hence consent is never directed at a medical intervention as such, but rather at some proposition that describes an intended intervention. However, any intervention can be described in many different ways. Even in the easy cases, where competent patients consent to a procedure or treatment described in a certain way, they may not be aware of and may not consent to other true descriptions of the same intervention, or of its more obvious effects. This can be the case even when the second description is entailed by the first, or when it refers to an obvious consequence of the state of affairs described by the first.

So propositional attitudes are opaque. A person may know or understand or hope that x, but not know or understand or hope that y, even where x entails y. A patient may consent to an intervention, and the intervention as described may entail or

bring about certain conditions, yet the patient may not consent to those conditions since he or she may not grasp the entailment relation or the causal connection. For example, a parent may consent to the removal of tissues from their dead child, and the undifferentiated reference to tissues will cover entire organs; however, the parent may not know that this is so, and be upset to discover that entire organs were removed on the basis of general consent to the removal of tissues.

Because propositional attitudes are always opaque, the basic difficulties of informed consent procedures cannot be reliably eliminated by making information more available or consent procedures easier to follow. For unless the information is actually understood by those whose informed consent is requested, genuine consent will not stretch to the relevant proposition. This difficulty is ubiquitous within the central debates of medical ethics, although barely discussed (O'Neill 2002b).

14.3 Explicit or implied? Specific or generic?

These difficulties have been heightened rather than resolved by recent attempts to improve informed consent procedures. Two supposed improvements are often advocated, and raise particular difficulties. The first demands that all consent should be explicit, rather than implied; the second that it be specific rather than generic.

The distinction between explicit and implied consent contrasts ways of consenting. Explicit consent typically relies on documents, signatures, and formal statements; it may require witnesses who confirm that proper procedures for consenting have been followed. The formal procedures are typically designed to create enduring records, thereby reducing later uncertainty about the consent given, and perhaps forestalling dissatisfaction, complaint, or litigation. Patients who consent explicitly to proposed interventions thereby accept that they cannot later claim that they were injured or wronged, and that they will not have grounds for complaint or litigation.

By contrast, implied consent is inferred from a patient's action. For example, agreement to blood being taken or to having an injection is standardly signified by extending one's arm for the doctor to take the blood or give the injection. No documentation of the consent is required. It would be possible—but laborious—to replace the implied consent that is currently seen as sufficient in these and similar cases with explicit consent procedures. It would be possible—but strenuous—to introduce explicit consent procedures for the most minor and routine of medical interventions. However much we introduce additional explicit procedures and consent forms for interventions that are now performed on the basis of implied consent, explicit consent always relies on background understandings that remain implicit. The longest and most complex consent form cannot include a complete description of everything that will be done. Much is taken as understood, and consent based on those understandings can only be implied. No programme for replacing implied with explicit consent can be complete.

The distinction between specific and generic consent applies to the propositions to which consent is given, rather than to processes of consenting. For example, consent may be given to the removal of tissues, or alternatively to the removal of a specific sort of tissue, or even to the removal of tissue for a specific use, such as diagnosis, or as part of a cancer treatment or post mortem to determine the cause of death. The descriptions to which consent is given are always incomplete. We can always add more detail. So those who believe that informed consent should be highly specific need to explain how specific it has to be to constitute ethically adequate informed consent. Answering this question may be no easier than answering the pseudo-question 'How long is a piece of string?'.

These problems are not 'merely theoretical'. They surface and create practical problems wherever data protection issues arise, in secondary data analyses, and in the use of tissues for comparative study. If personal information is to be 'processed' (obtained, recorded, processed, sorted, used) only in accordance with the consent of those to whom it pertains (the 'data subjects'), then it will constantly turn out that if the consent obtained is sufficiently specific to permit a certain use, it will also be sufficiently specific to preclude other uses.

Similarly, if tissues and information from past patients are to be studied for purposes that could not have been anticipated, they must be studied without specific consent, since such consent could not in principle have been requested or given at the relevant time. The problem is not merely that in the past consent procedures were too lax, and that the relevant consents were not obtained, or not recorded with sufficient clarity (although that was often the case). The problem is deeper, indeed irresolvable, because many valuable purposes could not have been anticipated at the time that tissues were removed and stored. For example, nobody could tell in advance when information and tissues obtained in the course of treating past patients will turn out to be useful for unanticipated research. Both clinical information and tissue samples pertaining to deceased patients may later turn out to be vital for reaching a better understanding of new diseases. When the first patient with Creutzfeldt–Jakob disease (vCJD) died, the only way in which pathologists could determine whether this was a new disease was by comparing their brain tissue with samples taken from patients who had died of CJD over many decades in many countries. Tissues and information from those who died in the 1918 influenza epidemic may yet prove valuable in studying emerging diseases (Gamblin, S. J. *et al.* 2004). It is difficult to see how secondary data analysis of this sort can proceed if access to tissue samples from and data pertaining to past patients, their treatment and their clinical outcomes cannot be consulted without specific prior consent to such studies. Although the incidence of disease could be monitored on the basis of collecting deidentified data, linked data are needed for all more elaborate forms of retrospective study and public health research. Specific consent requirements undermine secondary data analysis in medical and other areas of inquiry; they would close down epidemiology.

However, a claim that specific consent is ethically required for retrospective study of linked patient information and tissues is neither intuitive nor plausible—provided that standard safeguards such as the approval of ethics committees and anonymization are in place. What would we think of a patient who asks his doctor how he knows that a medicine will prove helpful, is told that it helped nearly all patents with same condition, accepts the treatment but then refuses consent to the further study of information—even anonymized information—about the clinical outcome in his own case?

14.4 Public health and public goods

There are further and more general reasons for rejecting the current tendency to suppose that informed consent procedures are the touchstone of ethically acceptable medical provision. One of the most significant is that informed consent procedures are inapplicable whenever the goods or benefits to be provided are public goods. Certain types of goods—consumer goods, clinical care—can be provided for individuals, and their provision can in principle be made contingent on individual consent. The difficulties that informed consent requirements raise may prove irresolvable in some cases, and resolvable in others. By contrast, if public goods are provided for any, they have to be provided for many. Some types of public good must be provided (or not provided) for whole populations; others may be provided (or not provided) for more restricted groups. For present purposes I leave these differences aside, to make the simple point that the provision of public goods cannot be made contingent on individual consent. For example, road safety, food safety, water safety, safe medicines, and measures that protect against infection cannot be tailored to individual choice. Because there are no obligations to do the impossible ('ought implies can'), informed consent cannot be ethically required for the provision of public goods, including public heath measures.

The implications of these thoughts about public goods are wider than may at first seem to be the case. For example, clinical care itself has to be provided to meet standards and formats that are also largely fixed and uniform, and so cannot be treated as a matter for informed consent. The scaffolding of professional training, of institutional structures, of public funding, of physical facilities are all public goods. The public provision of healthcare can reflect democratic process, and thereby certain forms of collective choice: but its basic structures cannot be geared to individual choice. Unavoidably there are large areas of medical ethics in which informed consent can play no part, or at most a minor part. What then are the appropriate ethical and other normative issues in these areas of medical ethics?

14.5 Health and justice

The ethical reasoning most commonly used in medical ethics focusses on transactions between individual professionals and individual patients, or between individual professionals and individual research subjects. Individualistic approaches are not likely to be useful for analysing ethical questions about the provision of public goods, such as public health provision. However, it may seem that theories of justice will also provide an inappropriate account of the normative reasoning most relevant to the provision of public goods, or to public health ethics. Most uses of theories of justice in healthcare ethics have addressed distributive issues, such as the just distribution of clinical care. Discussions of healthcare allocation decisions—of rationing—are discussions of the just distribution of a good that can be made contingent on individual choice. Theories of distributive justice also fail to address the distinctive ethical questions that arise in providing public goods, so are not helpful for public health ethics.

But there is more to justice than distributive justice. All theories of justice also address the justification of compulsion, and in particular the justification of the forms of compulsion on which any legal order depends. There are many differing theories of justice, but by way of illustration I shall instance one theory, because it gives a particularly large—supposedly maximal—role to individual liberty and so to individual consent procedures. This theory is John Stuart Mill's form of liberalism, especially as developed in On Liberty. I choose Mill's account of justice not because I assume or argue that it is more plausible than other accounts, but because he explicitly opposes compulsion except in very limited circumstances, and so provides a particularly severe standard for judging legitimate compulsion. Mill famously claimed that, the sole end for which mankind are warranted, individually or collectively, in interfering with the liberty of any of their number is self-protection. (Mill, J. S. 1859)

Compulsion, on this view, is permitted only where needed in order to protect others: it is unjust unless needed to prevent harm to others. Public health provision is an obvious area where Mill's arguments are relevant, since compulsion may be needed to prevent individual action that might harm others' health.

Prevention of transmission of disease is a central case for Mill's justification of compulsion. Given the death rate from SARS and the seriousness of the illness, Mill would view it as legitimate to make certain forms of action or treatment compulsory. The harms that may arise when the risk of transmission is moderately high, and the risk of death for those who succumb high for some age groups create a strong case for collective self-protection. Depending on the gravity of the risk, it might be permissible to institute mandatory monitoring of those who may have been exposed, mandatory vaccination (if a vaccine is developed), restrictions on free movement, or quarantine. Similarly, where vaccination is safe and effective, Mill's argument would suggest that it could legitimately be made compulsory in order to produce the herd immunity that protects vulnerable individuals who cannot (yet) be vaccinated. Making public health measures such as these compulsory would hardly have seemed controversial a century ago. It has come to seem controversial on the basis of an illusory assumption that all medical provision, and with it public health provision, can be organized on the basis of informed consent of individuals. It cannot.

Of course, there are always difficulties in judging how great a risk is, and in deciding which forms of compulsion are most effective and most readily justified in a particular case. Such issues can only be resolved on a case-by-case basis, using the right expertise and the right information. Often there are deficits in information and in expertise, as with the many uncertainties about the mode of transmission and likely spread of vCJD, and other new transmissible diseases. But where information and expertise point to the likelihood of harm to others there are, even on a very strong liberal account of justice, no good ethical arguments to forbid all compulsion. To the contrary, appeals to individual consent do not offer a coherent, let alone an acceptable, way of approaching public health provision. 'Salus populi suprema lex' is not an obsolete thought (Cicero 1928).

CHAPTER 15

What have we learnt from SARS?

Robin A. Weiss and Angela R. McLean

15.1 Summary

With outbreaks of infectious disease emerging from animal sources, we have learned to expect the unexpected. We were and are expecting a new influenza A pandemic, but no one predicted the emergence of an unknown coronavirus (CoV) as a deadly human pathogen. Thanks to the preparedness of the international network of influenza researchers and laboratories, the cause of severe acute respiratory syndrome (SARS) was rapidly identified, but there is no room for complacency over the global or local management of the epidemic in terms of public health logistics. The human population was lucky that only a small proportion of infected persons proved to be highly infectious, and that they did not become so before they felt ill. These were the features that helped to make the outbreak containable. The next outbreak of another kind of transmissible disease may well be quite different.

Since SARS was first recognized as something new and threatening, we have learned a tremendous amount about the disease—the causative virus, its transmission dynamics, and the collateral damage to local life and economy arising out of the fear and stress that SARS engendered. In bringing together authors from diverse disciplines who experienced the raw face of SARS as the story unfolded, this book enables us to reflect upon the dangers and logistics of an unexpected, previously unknown infectious disease with high mortality. Fortunately, SARS remained an outbreak rather than maturing into a pandemic, although we acknowledge the estimated 8098 cases of illness and mourn the 774 people who have died from SARS.

In this concluding chapter, we consider that although many of the lessons learned are specific to SARS, others apply more generally to epidemic infectious diseases. So why did SARS appear where and when it did? Whereas avian influenza and SARS have a Chinese origin, we should recall that in recent history other disease outbreaks usually of zoonotic origin have occurred on all continents: AIDS came 'out of Africa', BSE/vCJD is a truly British achievement, hantavirus pulmonary syndrome first appeared in the United States (as did Legionnaires' disease) and later in South America, and fruit bats (flying foxes) gave rise to hendravirus and nipahvirus in Australia and Malaysia, respectively. Rich or poor, North, South, East, or West, the lesson is that novel infectious diseases can appear anywhere (Weiss 2001).

As to why SARS arose in China at this time, the particular reasons discussed by Diana Bell and co-authors in Chapter 9 relate to the increasing popularity of exotic foods, in this case civet cats (viverrids). We still do not know what the natural reservoir species of this CoV is, but the importation, holding together, and rearing of so many species of viverrids and also one canid and one mustelid allowed its amplification and transfer to humans to occur. The rapidly expanding popularity of such animal foods in recent years as the Guangzhong population became more urbanized and increasingly wealthy may well explain why SARS is an early twenty-first-century disease, although sporadic human cases may have occurred in earlier times. While this interesting footnote of local culinary predilection to eat civet cats may explain this particular outbreak, the lesson of SARS for newly transmissible diseases in general is spelt out by Tony McMichael (Chapter 2) in surveying the pace of ecological and environmental change that brings about new animal–human interfaces, often where humans live densely and hence may provide conditions for onward transmission.

Changing patterns of human ecology and behaviour affect two, distinct steps in the development of a new transmissible disease. The first is altering the opportunity for animal-to-human transfer. Thus the more interspecies contacts occur, the greater the risk of zoonotic infection. The relatively high proportion of civet cat handlers and exotic food restaurateurs who have serum antibodies that react or cross-react to the SARS-CoV indicates that the zoonotic transfer of a related, less virulent virus may occur far more frequently than the adaptation of such a virus to onward transmission among humans. The close phylogenetic relationship of SARS-CoV genomes described by Eddie Holmes (Chapter 3) further indicates that the outbreak which went on to spread internationally had a point source, whereas the viral genomes among the civet cats appear to be more diverse. However, evidence is emerging that non-symptomatic SARS-related CoV infection may have travelled as far as Hong Kong before the disease outbreak (Zheng *et al.* 2004).

The second ecological factor is the opportunity for onward spread once a human has become infected. For every new pandemic like AIDS and 1918/1919 influenza, there are probably thousands of 'failed' transfers. These zoonoses include those that are inapparent, where infection does not result in pathogenesis, and those that may be fatal but are not usually transmissible between humans, such as rabies, or the 1997 H5N1 avian influenza outbreak in Hong Kong (for H5N1 in 2004 it was too early to tell at that time of writing, but its spread among chickens is already far more widespread, and the case reports of human transmission more ominous). So far, local outbreaks of Ebola virus and Lassa disease in Africa have petered out. Like SARS, infection with Ebola carries a particular exposure hazard for family and professional healthcarers, although there is no evidence of respiratory transmission. SARS was more mobile across our global village, perhaps only because of the greater frequency of international

air travel from southern China and Hong Kong than from central Africa. Dirk Brockmann (Chapter 11) uses probabilistic modelling to predict the intercontinental transfer of future emerging infections and how important it will be to respond rapidly in a focussed way in order to prevent their global spread.

Putting these two steps together generates a pathway to emergence in which new variants arise, occasionally infect individuals, and more infrequently still become capable of onward transmission from one person to another. Influenza is our best understood example of this iterative probing of the opportunities for emergence. Robin Bush (Chapter 4) describes how understanding the recent evolution of influenza teaches us general lessons about the emergence of novel infections. Frightening though SARS has been, it turned out to be controllable through careful containment of cases. Malik Peiris (Chapter 6) points out that this was only possible because SARS patients do not become highly infectious until after they are symptomatic. This is in direct contrast to influenza and many other infections where the burden of infectiousness largely precedes the onset of symptoms. By quantifying the relationships between time-to-infectiousness and time-to-disease Roy Anderson and colleagues (Chapter 10) classify infections into those that can and those that cannot be controlled through the isolation of cases.

Thus the differences between influenza and SARS may teach us more than their similarities do. Influenza infections will tend to create other cases before the index case is symptomatic; the influenza pandemic that we fear will have higher transmission rates than were seen in the 2003 SARS epidemic. What they share is direct transmission and a short incubation period. Some of the scariest emerging infections are those with long incubation periods, because for those, by the time the first cases are recognized, many infections have been generated and the logistics of control are correspondingly more difficult (Table 15.1). By the time AIDS was recognized as a novel disease, it was already spreading out of control in urban regions of the rich and poor world. By the time BSE was identified as more than just a few extra sick cows, it had spread across the United Kingdom

Table 15.1 Emerging infections classified by their infectiousness and incubation period.

Infectiousness, R_0	Incubation period from infection to disease	
	Short (days or weeks)	Long (years)
High	Influenza A	BSE
Low	SARS	HIV/AIDS

Notes: SARS was a frightening reminder of how quickly a novel infectious disease can emerge and spread. However, its short incubation period meant that the problem was recognized before infection had become widespread. Some of the difficulties of dealing with BSE and AIDS have been caused by the widespread dissemination of infection before the first cases were even recognized, a direct result of their long incubation periods. (See Anderson *et al.* chapter 10, this volume; Ferguson *et al.* 1999).

and abroad. Thus there are several dimensions to the classification of emergent infections: more or less transmissible, early versus late infectiousness, short or long periods between infection and disease. Viewed in such a light, SARS might almost be classified as 'easy' to manage.

The rapidity with which a new epidemic disease can spread raises questions over the balance of freedom of action of the individual and freedom from infection of the community at large. Onora O'Neill (Chapter 14) points out that it was easier to manage the SARS epidemic in a more controlled society with a strong sense of community, as in China, than in more individualistic, liberal democracies as in the West. All the same, the early phase of the SARS epidemic in Guangzhong province was poorly controlled in public health terms. The reasons were partly as discussed by Nanshan Zhong (Chapter 5), that SARS was not initially distinguished from a concurrent, more widespread influenza epidemic in Guangzhong; and partly the slowness of public health staff to realize that something new was afoot, and their initial reluctance to alert national authorities to the situation, thus abetting the spread of SARS to Beijing.

An important lesson learned in China, at the price of the resignations of the health minister and the mayor of Beijing, was the need for transparency and communication. Once it became aware of SARS, the World Health Organization (WHO) swung into gear to manage what rapidly became

an international outbreak as described by David Heymann (Chapter 12). The WHO officer in Hanoi, Dr Carlo Urbani, sadly succumbed to SARS but not before he had alerted the world to the gravity of the situation. Even before the causative agent of SARS was identified, as Roy Anderson points out (Chapter 10), the pattern of transmission was being analysed, and models of best containment began to evolve. On the other hand, Robert Maunder (Chapter 13) analyses the psychological stress to exposed healthcare workers who did not know if they were incubating SARS and who wished to spare their families from infection. They came to be regarded by some, not so much as heroes but as 'lepers' in their midst.

Perhaps the greatest achievement during the SARS outbreak was the rapid and magnificent effort of infectious disease laboratories to isolate and characterize the SARS coronavirus (Lingappa 2004), resulting in three groups in Hong Kong, Germany, and North America identifying the same agent. Malik Peiris (Chapter 6) describes how the virus came to light during the hectic days of the Hong Kong outbreak, Ab Osterhaus (Chapter 7) relates how it was possible to use Koch's postulates to prove the coronavirus guilty of causing SARS, and Maria Zambon (Chapter 8) illustrates how quickly sensitive and specific diagnostic methods were devised to determine who was infected by the SARS-CoV. This combined effort would not have been possible if the investigators had waited to receive specific funds to tackle SARS; rather, they diverted influenza funding urgently to explore this new emergency. Moreover, they could not have made such excellent progress if there had not been a pre-existing network of influenza surveillance and reference laboratories, and a rapid and open means of exchange of information and materials between them, and above all, a sense of trust and mutual endeavour.

The identification of the SARS-CoV rapidly led to the cloning and sequencing of the entire genome, and the expression of recombinant antigens for use in diagnostic tests. This knowledge has also led to candidate vaccines for immunization to protect against SARS-CoV infection. Promising results have been obtained with DNA based vaccines encoding the nucleocapsid protein or the envelope spike protein (Kim *et al.* 2004; Yang *et al.* 2004) and recombinant vaccines where the gene for the viral spike protein (S) is incorporated into adenovirus or vaccinia virus vectors (Gao *et al.* 2003; Bisht *et al.* 2004). However, it is crucial that the experimental study of the SARS-CoV does not itself lead to new outbreaks of infection from laboratory sources. It is disturbing that in three separate incidents in Taipei, Singapore, and Beijing laboratory personnel have become infected. In the most recent lapse of laboratory containment, the index patient, a graduate student, infected her mother who died and a nurse who in turn spread the infection to several members of her family (Normile 2004), and some 2000 had to be quarantined. Provided that laboratory safety protocols are rigorously followed, such infections should not occur, and the WHO is considering an international register of all laboratories that hold SARS-CoV. Much laboratory research can be undertaken without the need to handle the pathogen itself. For instance, replication-defective retroviral vectors bearing the SARS spike protein can be substituted for SARS-CoV in order to characterize cell entry by the virus and to conduct serum neutralization studies (Simmons *et al.* 2004).

A lesson that requires to be continually taught is the need for novel means of surveillance, cooperation between the public health and academic sectors, and the provision of enough trained scientists with the time and curiosity to experiment improving tests and keeping abreast of animal and human virology and microbiology in 'peacetime', in order to rise to the challenge in emergency. For example, the dearth of professional clinical virologists in the United Kingdom, parallels the erosion of state veterinary virologists highlighted after the 2001 epidemic of foot-and-mouth disease (Royal Society 2002). When it comes to training and employing the next generation of infectious disease specialists, it would appear that the reproductive rate, R_0, is less than 1.

In the end, if it is the end, fewer than 1000 persons died from SARS, which makes it a minor cause of disease viewed on the global scale (Fig. 15.1). However, another lesson learned from SARS is how much greater the social and economic impact of the outbreak has been than one would

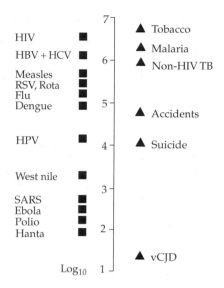

Figure 15.1 Natural weapons of mass destruction: a 'Richter' scale for global viral diseases measured as approximate numbers of deaths in 2003. This is a snap-shot picture in time; for instance, the estimated yearly death toll of HIV has risen 10,000-fold in the past 20 years, whereas polio has fallen approximately 1000-fold thanks to successful vaccination policies. Vaccines—weapons of mass protection—led to the eradication or reduction of smallpox, yellow fever, polio, and MMR. HIV, human immunodeficient virus; HBV, hepatitis B virus; HCV, hepatitis C virus; RSV, respiratory syncytial virus; HPV, human papilloma virus; SARS, severe acute respiratory syndrome; TB, tuberculosis; vCJD, variant Creutzfeldt-Jakob disease; MMR, measles, mumps, and rubella. (Adapted from Hale et al. 2001).

have expected from calculating the actual number of deaths or days off work through sickness. Human society has had much reason to fear pestilence in the past (Weiss 2001) and in March 2003, it was not yet clear whether SARS was to be the 'big one'. Moreover, suppose SARS arose when it did in the Middle East rather than Far East? The inevitable conspiracy theories on deliberate release would have been rife and might have been used as a further excuse for war, though it might have deterred the advance of an occupying force.

Our main conclusion from the multidisciplinary discussion meeting of SARS presented in this book, is that humankind has had a lucky escape. Suppose that the SARS coronavirus (SARS-CoV) became readily transmissible from person-to-person before people became seriously ill with disease, as is the case with influenza A? Suppose that a much higher proportion of infected people served as 'superspreaders'? We do not yet know which human predispositions or genetic polymorphisms determine susceptibility to severe disease following SARS-CoV infection, or determine superspreader status, which is not synonymous with mortality. Perhaps it will prove to be related to the recently identified cell surface receptor for the virus (Li *et al* 2003*b*; Wang *et al* 2004), or perhaps to the infected person's immune constitution. If the latter, suppose the virus had flown from Hong Kong to Durban instead of Toronto? It is a city of similar size but without a similar health infrastructure, and with a significant proportion of its inhabitants immunocompromised on account of HIV-1 infection. Then Africa could have become endemic for SARS by now. Epidemiologists and public health experts sometimes frown upon us for indulging in such 'What if?' scenarios. However, modelling what has not yet happened, but might unfold next time, is surely part of contingency planning and preparedness.

References

Alaszewski, A. and Horlick-Jones, T. 2003. How can doctors communicate information about risk more effectively?, *BMJ* **327**, 728–731.

Amato, G. *et al.* 1999. A new species of muntjac *Muntiacus putaoensis* (Artiodactyla: Cervidae) from northern Myanmar. *Anim. Conserv.* **2**, 1–7.

Anderson, R. M. and May, R. M. 1991. *Infectious diseases of humans: dynamics and control.* Oxford Science Publications.

Anon. 1994. 1994 Plague—international team of experts, India. *Wkly. Epidem. Rec.* **69**, 321–322.

Anon. 2003*a*. Influenza A(H5N1), Hong Kong Special Administrative Region of China. *Wkly. Epidem. Rec.* **78**, 49–50.

Anon. 2003*b*. Acute respiratory syndrome, China. *Wkly. Epidem. Rec.* 2003, **78**, 41.

Anon. 2003*c*. SARS—*Chronology of events*. Ottawa: Health Canada, Population and Public Health Branch.

Anon. 2004*a*. China: towards 'xiaokang', but still living dangerously. *Lancet* **363**, 409.

Anon. 2004*b*. Indo-Burma Hotspot www.biodiversityhotspots.org/xp/Hotspots/indo_burma

Antia, R. *et al.* 2003. The role of evolution in the emergence of infectious diseases. *Nature* **426**, 658–610.

AOG. 2003. OAG Worldwide Limited, Bedfordshire, United Kingdom.

Baranowski, E. *et al.* 2001. Evolution of cell recognition by viruses. *Science* **292**, 1102–1105.

Barnes, R. 2002. The bushmeat boom and bust in west and central Africa. *Oryx.* **36**, 236–242.

Bell, G. 1997. *Selection: the mechanism of evolution.* London: Chapman and Hall.

Bennett, E. L. and Rao, M. 2002. Wild meat consumption in Asian tropical forest countries; is this a glimpse of the future for Africa? In *Links between biodiversity, conservation, livelihoods and food security: the sustainable use of wild species for meat* (eds. S. Mainka and M. Trivedi) Switzerland: IUCN, Gland, pp. 39–44.

Berger, A. *et al.* 2004. Severe acute respiratory syndrome (SARS)-paradigm of an emerging viral infection, *J. Clin. Virol.* **29(1)**, 13–22.

Bernoulli, D. 1760. Essai d'une nouvelle analyse de la mortalité causée par la petite véerole et des avantages de l'inoculation pour la prévenir. *Mém. Math. Phys. Acad. Roy. Sci., Paris*, page 1.

Bisht, H. *et al.* 2004. Severe acute respiratory syndrome coronavirus spike protein expressed by attenuated vaccinia virus protectively immunizes mice. *Proc. Natl. Acad. Sci. USA* **101**, 6641–6646.

Bowen-Jones, E. *et al.* 2003. Economic commodity or environmental crisis? An interdisciplinary approach to analysing the bushmeat trade in central and west Africa. *Area* **35**, 390–402.

Breiman, R. F. *et al.* 2003. Role of China in the quest to define and control severe acute respiratory syndrome. *Emerg. Infect. Dis.* **9**, 1037–1041.

Brooks, T. M. *et al.* 2002. Habitat loss and extinction in the hotspots of biodiversity. *Conserv. Biol.* **16**, 909–923.

Bush, R. M. *et al.* 1999. Positive selection on the H3 hemagglutinin gene of human influenza virus A. *Mol. Biol. Evol.* **16**, 1457–1465.

Bush, R. M. *et al.* 2000. Effects of passage history and sampling bias on phylogenetic reconstruction of human influenza A evolution. *Proc. Natl. Acad. Sci. USA* **97**, 6974–6980.

Bush, R. M. *et al.* 2001. Predicting influenza evolution: the impact of terminal and egg-adapted mutations. In *Options for the control of influenza*, Vol. 4 (ed. A. D. M. E. Osterhaus). Amsterdam: Elsevier, pp. 147–153.

Callaghan, P. and Morrisey, J. 1993. Social support and health: a review. *J. Adv. Nursing* **18**, 203–10.

Centers for Disease Control and Prevention 2003. Prevalence of IgG antibody to SARS-associated coronavirus in animal traders: Guangdong Province, China, 2003. *Morb. Mortal. Wkly. Rep.* **17**, 986–987.

Centers for Disease Control and Prevention 2003. Update: Outbreak of severe acute respiratory syndrome—worldwide, 2003. *Morb. Mortal. Wkly. Rep.* **52**, 241.

Chan, A. O. M. and Huak, C. Y. 2004. Psychological impact of the 2003 severe acute respiratory syndrome outbreak on health care workers in a medium size regional general hospital in Singapore, *Occupat. Med.* **54**, 190–196.

Chan, K. H. *et al.* 2004. Detection of SARS coronavirus in patients with suspected SARS. *Emerg. Infect. Dis.* **10**, 294–299.

Chan-Yeung, M. and Yu, W. C. 2003. Outbreak of severe acute respiratory syndrome in Hong Kong special administrative region: case report. *Br. Med. J.* **326**, 850–852.

Charleston, M. A. and Robertson, D. L. 2002. Preferential host switching by primate lentiviruses can account for phylogenetic similarity with the primate phylogeny. *Syst. Biol.* **51**, 528–535.

Chow, P. K. H. *et al.* 2004. Healthcare worker seroconversion in SARS outbreak. *Emerg. Infect. Dis.* **10**, 249–250.

Chua, K. *et al.* 2002. Anthropogenic deforestation, El Nino and the emergence of Nipah virus in Malaysia. *Malay. J. Pathol.* **24**, 15–21.

Chua, K. B. *et al.* 2000. Nipah virus: a recently emergent deadly paramyxovirus. *Science* **288**, 1432–1435.

Cicero, M. T. 1928. De Legibus, III, iii, 8. In Cicero, M.T., *De Re Publica, De Legibus*, tr. Clinton Walker Keyes, Loeb Classical Library.

Claas, E. C. and Osterhaus, A. D. M. E. 1998. New clues to the emergence of flu pandemics. *Nature Med.* **4**, 1122–1123.

Claas, E. C. *et al.* 1998. Human influenza A H5N1 virus related to a highly pathogenic avian influenza virus. *Lancet* **351**, 472–477.

Cleaveland, S. *et al.* 2001. Diseases of humans and their domestic mammals: pathogen characteristics, host range and the risk of emergence. *Phil. Trans. R. Soc. Lond. B* **356**, 991–999.

Cohen, A. 2003. Urban unfinished business. *Int. J. Environ. Hlth Res.* **13**, S29–S36.

Compton, J. and Quang, L.H. 1998. *Borderline: An Assessment of Wildlife Trade in Vietnam*. Hanoi, Vietnam: WWF Indochina Programme, 37 pp.

Cox, N. J. and Bender, C. A. 1995. The molecular epidemiology of influenza viruses. *Seminars Virol.* **6**, 359–370.

Cox, N. *et al.* 1993. Evolution of hemagglutinin in epidemic variants and selection of vaccine viruses. In *Options for the control of influenza*, Vol. 2 (eds. C. Hannoun, A. P. Kendal, H. D. Klenk, and F. L. Ruben). Amsterdam: Elsevier, pp. 223–230.

Crotty, S. *et al.* 2001. RNA virus error catastrophe: direct test by using ribavirin. *Proc. Natl. Acad. Sci. USA* **98**, 6895–6900.

Cuevas, J. M. *et al.* 2002. Molecular basis of adaptive convergence in experimental populations of RNA viruses. *Genetics* **162**, 533–542.

Culley, A. I. *et al.* 2003. High diversity of unknown picorna-like viruses in the sea. *Nature* **424**, 1054–1057.

Darwin, C. R. 1839. Journal and remarks, 1832–1836. Quoted in F. W. Nicholas and J. M. Nicholas 2002. *Charles Darwin in Australia*. Cambridge: Cambridge University Press, pp. 30–31.

Daszak, P. *et al.* 2001. Anthropogenic environmental change and the emergence of infectious diseases in wildlife. *Acta Trop.* **78**, 103–116.

Daubin, V. *et al.* 2003. Phylogenetics and the cohesion of bacterial genomes. *Science* **301**, 829–832.

Davis, S. D. *et al.* 1995. *Centres of plant diversity: a guide and strategy for their conservation. Volume 2: Asia, Australasia and the Pacific*. Cambridge, UK: IUCN Publications Unit.

de Jong, J. C. *et al.* 1997. A pandemic warning? *Nature* **389**, 554.

de Jong, J. C. *et al.* 2000. Influenza virus: a master of metamorphosis. *J. Infect.* **40**, 218–228.

DeFilippis, V. R. and Villarreal, L. P. 2000. An introduction to the evolutionary ecology of viruses. In *Viral ecology* (ed. C. J. Hurst), Academic Press, pp. 126–208.

Department of Health Hong Kong: Investigation report an outbreak of severe acute respiratory syndrome at Amoy Gardens Kowloon Bay, Hong Kong, Department of Health; Hong Kong Special Administrative Region, April 2003.

Diamond, J. 1997. *Guns, germs and steel*. London: Vintage.

Dinerstein, E. *et al.* 1999. A workbook for conducting biological assessments and developing biodiversity visions for ecoregion-based conservation.1: terrestrial ecoregions. WWF-US Conservation Science Program, Washington DC.

Dobson, A. P. and Carper, E. R. 1996. Infectious diseases and human population history. *Bioscience* **46**, 115–126.

Donnelly, C. A. *et al.* 2003. Epidemiological determinants of spread of causal agent of severe acute respiratory syndrome in Hong Kong. *Lancet* **361**, 1761–1766.

Drake, J. W. *et al.* 1998. Rates of spontaneous mutation. *Genetics* **148**, 1667–1686.

Drosten, C. *et al.* 2003. Identification of a novel coronavirus in patients with severe acute respiratory syndrome. *N. Engl. J. Med.* **348(20)**, 1967–1976.

Dubos, R. 1980. *The wooing of earth*. New York: Scribners.

Duckworth, J. W. *et al.* 1999. Wildlife in Lao PDR:1999 Status Report. Vientiane: IUCN-The World Conservation Union/Wildlife Conservation Society/Centre for Protected Areas and Watershed Management. Vientiane.

Dung, V. V. *et al.* 1994. Discovery and conservation of the Vu Quang Ox in Vietnam. *Oryx* **28**, 16–21.

Eickmann, M. *et al.* 2003. Phylogeny of the SARS coronavirus. *Science* **302**, 1504–1505.

Eigen, M. 1987. New concepts for dealing with the evolution of nucleic acids. *Cold Spring Harb. Symp. Quant. Biol.* **52**, 307–320.

Eigen, M. 1996. On the nature of virus quasispecies. *Trends Microbiol.* **4**, 216–218.

Emery, S. L. *et al.* 2004. Real-Time reverse transcription-polymerase chain reaction assay for SARS-associated coronavirus. *Emerg. Infect. Dis.* **10**, 311–316.

Engelthaler, D. M. *et al.* 1999. Climatic and environmental patterns associated with hantavirus pulmonary syndrome, Four Corners region, United States. *Emerg. Infect. Dis.* **5**, 87–94.

Fa, J. E. *et al.* 2002. Bushmeat exploitation in tropical forests: an intercontinental comparison. *Conserv. Biol.* **16**, 232–237.

Fa, J. E. *et al.* 2003. Bushmeat and food security in the Congo Basin: linkages between wildlife and people's future. *Environ. Conserv.* **30**, 71–78.

Fa, J. E. *et al.* 2004. Hunting vulnerability, ecological characteristics and harvest rates of bushmeat species in Afrotropical forests. *Biol. Conser* **121**, 167–176.

Faden, R. and Beauchamp, T. 1986. *A history and theory of informed consent.* Oxford University Press.

Fanning, T. G. *et al.* 2002. 1917 avian influenza virus sequences suggest that the 1918 pandemic virus did not acquire its hemagglutinin directly from birds. *J. Virol.* **76**, 7860–7862.

Farmer, P. 1999, *Infections and inequalities. The modern plagues.* Berkeley, CA: University of California Press.

Felsenstein, J. 1978. Cases in which parsimony or compatibility methods will be positively misleading. *Syst. Zool.* **27**, 401–410.

Ferguson, N. M. *et al.* 1999. Estimation of the basic reproduction number of BSE: the intensity of transmission in British cattle. *Proc. R. Soc. Lond. B.* **266**, 23–32.

Ferguson, N. M. *et al.* 2001a. The foot and mouth epidemic in Great Britain: pattern of spread and impact of interventions. *Science* **292**, 1155–1160.

Ferguson, N. M. *et al.* 2001b. Transmission intensity and impact of control policies on the foot and mouth epidemic in Great Britain. *Nature* **413**, 542–548.

Ferguson, N. M. *et al.* 2004. Assessing the public health risk posed by the avian H5N1 influenza epidemic. *Science* **304**, 968–969.

Fineberg, H. and Wilson, M. 1996. Social vulnerability and death by infection. *N. Engl. J. Med.* **334**, 859–860.

Folkman, S. and Greer, S. 2000. Promoting psychological well-being in the face of serious illness: when theory, research and practice inform each other. *Psycho oncology* **9**, 11–19.

Fouchier, R. A. *et al.* 2003. Aetiology: Koch's postulates fulfilled for SARS virus. *Nature* **423**, 240.

Fraley, R. C. *et al.* 2002. An item response theory analysis of self-report measures of adult attachment. *J. Pers. Soc. Psychol.* **78(2)**, 350–365.

Fraser, C. *et al.* 2004. What makes an infectious disease outbreak controllable? *Proc. Natl. Acad. Sci. USA* **101**, 6146–6151.

Galea, S. *et al.* 2003. Trends of probable post-traumatic stress disorder in New York City after the September 11 terrorist attacks. *Am. J. Epidemiol.* **158(6)**, 514–524.

Galen, R. S. and Gambino, S. R. 1975. *Beyond normality: the predictive value and efficiency of medical diagnosis.* New York: Wiley.

Galvani, A. P. *et al.* 2003. Severe acute respiratory syndrome: temporal stability and geographic variation in case-fatality rates and doubling times. *Emerg. Infect. Dis.* **9**, 991–994.

Gamblin, S. J. *et al.* 2004. The structure and receptor-binding properties of the 1918 influenza hemagglutinin. *Science* **303**, 1838–1842.

Gao, F. *et al.* 1999. Origin of HIV-1 in the chimpanzee. *Pan troglodytes troglodytes. Nature* **397**, 436–441.

Gao, W. *et al.* 2003. Effects of a SARS-associated coronavirus vaccine in monkeys. *Lancet* **362**, 1895–1896.

Gardiner, C. W. 1985. *Handbook of stochastic methods.* Berlin: Springer Verlag.

Giao, P. M. *et al.* 1998. Description of *Muntiacus truongsonensis*, a new species of muntjac (Artiodactyla: Muntiacidae) from central Vietnam, and implications for conservation. *Anim. Conserv.* **1**, 61–68.

Gibbs, A. J. *et al.* 2004. The phylogeny of SARS coronavirus. *Arch. Virol.* **149**, 621–624.

Gibbs, M. J. *et al.* 2001. Recombination in the hemagglutinin gene of the 1918 'Spanish flu'. *Science* **293**, 1842–1845.

Glass, G. *et al.* 1995. Environmental risk factors for Lyme disease identified with geographical information systems. *Am. J. Public Hlth.* **85**, 944–948.

Grant, P. R. *et al.* 2003. Detection of SARS coronavirus in plasma by real-time RT-PCR. *N. Engl. J. Med.* **349**, 2468–2469.

Grenfell, B. T. *et al.* 2001. Travelling waves and spatial hierarchies in measles epidemics. *Nature* **414**, 716.

Guan, Y. *et al.* 1999. Molecular characterization of H9N2 influenza viruses: were they the donors of the 'internal' genes of H5N1 viruses in Hong Kong? *Proc. Natl. Acad. Sci. USA* **96**, 9363–9367.

Guan, Y. *et al.* 2003. Isolation and characterization of viruses related to the SARS Coronavirus from animals in southern China. *Science* **302**, 276–278.

Guan, Y. *et al.* 2004. Molecular epidemiology of the novel coronavirus that causes severe acute respiratory syndrome. *Lancet* **363**, 99–104.

Haagmans, B. L. *et al.* 2004. Pegylated interferonalpha protects type 1 pneumocytes against SARS coronavirus infection in macaques. *Nature Med.* **10**, 290–293.

Hahn, B. H. *et al.* 2000. AIDS as a zoonosis: scientific and public health implications. *Science* **287**, 607–614.

Hale, P. *et al.* 2001. Mission now possible for AIDS fund. *Nature* **412**, 271–272.

Hales, S. *et al.* 2002. Potential effect of population and climate changes on global distribution of dengue fever: an empirical model. *Lancet* **360**, 830–834.

Harvell, C. *et al.* 2002. Climate warming and disease risks for terrestrial and marine biota. *Science* **296**, 2158–2162.

Hayden, F. G. *et al.* 1998. Local and systemic cytokine responses during experimental human influenza A virus infection. Relation to symptom formation and host defense. *J. Clin. Invest.* **101**, 643–649.

He, J.-F. *et al.* 2004. Molecular evolution of the SARS coronavirus during the course of the SARS epidemic in China. *Science* **303**, 1666–1669.

Health Canada 2002. Global public health intelligence network. URL: www.cscw.ca/surveillance/projects/wyd/docs/Alert20020710.pdf

Health Canada 2003. *Canadian SARS Numbers* Available: www.hc-sc.gc.ca/pphb-dgspsp/sars-sras/cn-cc/numbers.html (accessed January 19, 2004), Ottawa.

Hearn, J. 2001. Unfair game – The bushmeat trade is wiping out large African mammals. *Sci. Amer.* **284**, 24–26.

Heymann, D. L. and Rodier, G. 2001. Hot spots in a wired world: WHO surveillance of emerging and re-emerging infectious diseases. *Lancet Infect. Dis.* **1**, 345–353.

Heymann, D. L. *et al.* 1999. Ebola hemorrhagic fever: lessons from Kikwit, Democratic Republic of the Congo. *J. Infect. Dis.* **179(Suppl.1)**, S283–S286.

Hien, T. T. *et al.* 2004. Avian influenza A (H5N1) in 10 patients in Vietnam. *N. Engl. J. Med.* **350**, 1179–1188.

Hillis, D. M. 1996. Inferring complex phylogenies. *Nature* **383**, 130–131.

Hoffmann, E. *et al.* 2000. Characterization of the influenza A virus gene pool in avian species in southern China: was H6N1 a derivative or a precursor of H5N1? *J. Virol.* **74**, 6309–6315.

Holmes, E. C. 2003. Patterns of intra- and inter-host nonsynonymous variation reveal strong purifying selection in dengue virus. *J. Virol.* **77**, 11296–11298.

Holmes, E. C. 2004. The phylogeography of human viruses. *Mol. Ecol.* **13**, 745–756.

Holmes, K. V. and Enjuanes, L. 2003. The SARS coronavirus: a postgenomic era. *Science* **300**, 1377–1378.

Horowitz, M. *et al.* 1979. Impact of event scale: a measure of subjective stress. *Psychosom. Med.* **41**, 209–218.

Horowitz, M. J. *et al.* 2000. Impact of event scale (IES), in *Handbook of Psychiatric Measures*, Task Force for the Handbook of Psychiatric Measures *et al.*, (eds.), American Psychiatric Publishing Group, Washington DC, 579–581.

Hsu, L. Y. *et al.* 2003. Severe acute respiratory syndrome (SARS) in Singapore: clinical features of index patient and initial contacts. *Emerg. Infect. Dis.* **9**, 713–717.

Huelsenbeck, J. P. *et al.* 2001. Bayesian inference of phylogeny and its impact on evolutionary biology. *Science* **294**, 2310–2314.

Hull, R. *et al.* 2000. Genetically modified plants and the 35S promoter: assessing the risks and enhancing the debate. *Microb. Ecol. Health Dis.* **12**, 1–5.

Hunter, J. J. and Maunder, R. G. 2001. Using attachment theory to understand illness behavior. *Gen. Hosp. Psychiatr.* **23**, 177–182.

IATA 2003. International Air Transport Association (IATA), Geneva, Switzerland.

Intergovernmental Panel on Climate Change (IPCC) 2001. *Climate Change 2001: the scientific basis: contribution of working group 1 to the third Assessment Report.* Cambridge: Cambridge University Press.

Jenkins, G. M. *et al.* 2002. Rates of molecular evolution in RNA viruses: a quantitative phylogenetic analysis. *J. Mol. Evol.* **54**, 152–161.

Jernigan, J. A. *et al.* 2004. Combining clinical and epidemiological features for early recognition of SARS. *Emerg. Infect. Dis.* **10**, 327–333.

Johnsen, B. *et al.* 1997. Post traumatic stress symptoms in non-exposed, victims and rescuers after an avalanche. *J. Trauma Stress* **10(133)**, 140.

Karl, T. and Trenberth, K. 2003. Modern global climate change. *Science* **302**, 1719–1723.

Kawaoka, Y. *et al.* 1989. Avian-to-human transmission of the PB1 gene of influenza A viruses in the 1957 and 1968 pandemics. *J. Virol.* **63**, 4603–4608.

Keeling, M. J. *et al.* 2001. Dynamics of the 2001 UK foot and mouth epidemic: stochastic dispersal in a heterogeneous landscape. *Science* **294**, 813–817.

Keeling, M. J. *et al.* 2003. Modelling vaccination strategies against foot-and-mouth disease. *Nature* **421**, 136–142.

Khan, A. S. *et al.* 1999. The re-emergence of Ebola hemorrhagic fever, Democratic Republic of the Congo, 1995. *J. Infect. Dis.* **179(Suppl.1)**, S76–S86.

Kim, T. W. *et al.* 2004. Generation and characterization of DNA vaccines targeting the nucleocapsid protein of severe acute respiratory syndrome coronavirus. *J. Virol.* **78**, 4638–4645.

Kishino, H. and Hasegawa, M. 1989. Evaluation of the maximum likelihood estimate of the evolutionary tree topologies from DNA sequence data, and the branching order of the hominoidea. *J. Mol. Evol.* **29**, 170–179.

Ksiazek, T. G. *et al.* 2003. A novel coronavirus associated with severe acute respiratory syndrome. *N. Engl. J. Med.* **348(20)**, 1953–1966.

Kuiken, T. *et al.* 2003*a*. Newly discovered coronavirus as the primary cause of severe acute respiratory syndrome. *Lancet* **362**, 263–270.

Kuiken, T. *et al.* 2003*b*. Emerging viral infections in a rapidly changing world. *Curr. Opin. Biotechnol.* **14**, 641–646.

Kuiken, T. *et al.* 2004. Experimental human metapneumovirus infection of cynomolgus macaques (*Macaca fascicularis*) results in virus replication in ciliated epithelial cells and pneumocytes with associated lesions throughout the respiratory tract. *Am. J. Pathol.* (in press).

Kuno, G. 1995. Review of the factors modulating dengue transmission. *Epidem. Rev.* **17**, 321–335.

Kuo, Y.-H. 2002. Extrapolation of correlation between 2 variables in 4 general medical journals. *JAMA* **287**, 2815–2817.

Lai, M. M. C. 1996. Recombination in large RNA viruses: coronaviruses. *Semin. Virol.* **7**, 381–388.

Lancee, W. J. *et al.* 2004. The acute traumatic impact of the SARS outbreak on hospital healthcare workers in Toronto. *Psychosom Med.* **66(1)**, A21.

Langer, W. L. 1964. The black death. *Sci. Am.* **2**, 114.

Lee, K. and Dodgson, R. 2000. Globalisation and cholera: implications for global governance. *Global Governance 2000* **6**, 213–236.

Lee, M. L. *et al.* 2003*a*. Use of quarantine to prevent transmission of severe acute respiratory syndrome—Taiwan, 2003. *MMWR* **52**, 680–683.

Lee, N. *et al.* 2003*b*. A major outbreak of severe acute respiratory syndrome in Hong Kong. *N. Engl. J. Med.* **348**, 1986–1994.

Leung, G. M. *et al.* 2004*a*. The epidemiology of severe acute respiratory syndrome (SARS) in the 2003 Hong Kong epidemic: analysis of all 1755 patients. *Ann. Internal Med.* **141**, 662–673.

Leung, G. M. *et al.* 2004*b*. SARS-CoV Antibody prevalence in all Hong Kong patient contacts. *Emerg. Infect. Dis.* **10**, 1653–1656.

Li, G. *et al.* 2003*a*. Profile of specific antibodies to the SARS-associated coronavirus. *N. Engl. J. Med.* **349**, 508–509.

Li, W. *et al.* 2003*b*. Angiotensin-converting enzyme 2 is a functional receptor for the SARS coronavirus. *Nature* **426**, 450–54.

Lindgren, E. and Gustafson, R. 2001. Tick-borne encephalitis in Sweden and climate change. *Lancet* **358**, 16–18.

Lingappa, J. 2004. Wresting SARS from uncertainty. *Emerg. Infect. Dis.* **10**, 167–170.

Lipsitch, M. *et al.* 2003. Transmission dynamics and control of severe acute respiratory syndrome. *Science* **300**, 1966–1970.

Lloyd-Smith, J. O. *et al.* 2003. Curtailing transmission of severe acute respiratory syndrome within a community and its hospital. *Proc. R. Soc. Lond. B* **270**, 1979–1989 (DOI 10.1098/rspb.2003.2481).

Low, D. E. 2004. Why SARS will not return: A polemic. *CMAJ* **170**, 68–69.

Low, D. E. and McGeer, A. 2003. SARS—one year later. *N. Engl. J. Med.* **349**, 2381–2382.

Lynch, M. *et al.* 1999. Salmonella tel-el-kebir and terrapins. *J. Infect.* **38**, 182–184.

Macdonald, D. 2001. *The new encyclopaedia of mammals.* Oxford: Oxford University Press.

Mahon, B. E. *et al.* 1997. An international outbreak of salmonella infections caused by alfalfa sprouts grown from contaminated seeds. *J. Infect. Dis. USA* **91**, 2395–2400.

Maiztegui, J. I. 1975. Clinical and epidemiological patterns of Argentine haemorrhagic fever. *Bull. WHO* **52**, 567–575.

Malpica, M. J. *et al.* 2002. The rate and character of spontaneous mutation in an RNA virus. *Genetics* **162**, 1505–1511.

Marra, M. A. *et al.* 2003. The genome sequence of the SARS-associated coronavirus. *Science* **300**, 1399–1404.

Martens W. J. M. *et al.* 1999. Climate change and future populations at risk of malaria. *Global Environ. Change* **9(Suppl.)**, S89–S107.

Martina, B. E. *et al.* 2003. Virology: SARS virus infection of cats and ferrets. *Nature* **425**, 915.

Matrosovich, M. N. *et al.* 1993. Probing of the receptor-binding sites of the H1 and H3 influenza A and influenza B virus hemagglutinins by synthetic and natural sialosides. *J. Virol.* **196**, 111–121.

Matthee, C. A. *et al.* 2004. A molecular supermatrix of the rabbits and hares (Leporidae) allows for five intercontinental exchanges during the Miocene. *Syst. Biol.* **53**, 433–447.

Maunder, R. G. and Hunter, J. J. 2001. Attachment and psychosomatic medicine: developmental contributions to stress and disease. *Psychosom Med.* **63**, 556–567.

Maunder, R. *et al.* 2003. The immediate psychological and occupational impact of the 2003 SARS outbreak in a teaching hospital. *CMAJ* **168**, 1245–1251.

Maynard Smith, J. and Szathmáry, E. 1995. *The major transitions of evolution.* W. H. Freeman and Co.

Mazzoni, R. *et al.* 2003. Emerging pathogen of wild amphibians in frogs (*Rana catesbeiana*) farmed for international trade. *Emerg. Infect. Dis.* **9**, 995–998.

McBride, F. 2003. Communicating during a crisis–the SARS story at Mount Sinai Hospital. *Hosp. Q.* **6(4)**, 51–53.

McGillis Hall, L. *et al.* 2003. 'Media portrayal of nurses' perspectives and concerns in the SARS crisis in Toronto. *J. Nurs. Scholar.* **35**, 211–216.

McLysaght, A. *et al.* 2002. Extensive genomic duplication during early chordate evolution. *Nat. Genet.* **31**, 200–204.

McLysaght, A. *et al.* 2003. Extensive gene gain associated with adaptive evolution of poxviruses. *Proc. Natl. Acad. Sci. USA* **100**, 14960–14965.

McMichael, A. J. 2001. *Human frontiers, environments and disease: past patterns, uncertain futures.* Cambridge: Cambridge University Press.

McMichael, A. J. 2002. Population, environment, disease, and survival: past patterns, uncertain futures. *Lancet* **359**, 1145–1148.

McMichael, A. J. *et al.* 2003. Global climate change. In: *Comparative quantification of health risks: global and regional burden of disease attributable to selected major risk factors* (eds., M. Ezzati, A. Lopez, A. Rodgers, and C. Murray). Geneva, World Health Organization.

McNeill, W. 1975. *Plagues and peoples.* Middlesex: Penguin.

Mill, J. S. 1989. On liberty, (1859). In *On liberty and other writings* (ed. S. Collini). Cambridge University Press, ch. 1, 13.

Milner-Gulland, E. J. *et al.* 2003. Wild meat: the bigger picture. *Trends Ecol. Evol.* **18**, 351–357

Mollison, D. 1991. The dependence of epidemic and population velocities on basic parameters. *Math. Biosci.* **107**, 255.

Monath, T. 1994. Dengue: the risk to developed and developing countries. *Proc. Natl. Acad. Sci. USA* **91**, 2395–2400.

Moore, P. *et al.* 1989. Intercontinental spread of an epidemic group A *Neisseria meningitidis* strain. *Lancet* **2**, 260–263.

Moroney, J. F. *et al.* 1998. Detection of chlamydiosis in a shipment of pet birds, leading to recognition of an outbreak of clinically mild psittacosis in humans. *Clin. Infect. Dis.* **26**, 1425–1429.

Morse, S. S. 1995. Factors in the emergence of infectious diseases. *Emerg. Infect. Dis.* **1**, 7–15.

Murray, J. D. 1993. *Mathematical biology.* New York: Springer-Verlag Berlin Heidelberg.

National Advisory Committee on SARS and Public Health. 2003. *Learning from SARS: Renewal of Public Health in Canada.* Government of Canada, Ottawa, Canada.

Neumann, G. *et al.* 2003. Reverse genetics for the control of avian influenza. *Avian Dis.* **47**, 882–887.

Ng, S. K. 2003. Possible role of an animal vector in the SARS outbreak at Amoy Gardens. *Lancet* **362**, 570–572.

Nicholls, J. M. *et al.* 2003. Lung pathology of fatal severe acute respiratory syndrome. *Lancet* **361**, 1773–1778.

Nickell, L. A. *et al.* 2004. Psychosocial impacts of SARS on hospital staff: Survey study of a large, tertiary health care institution in Toronto, Canada. *CMAJ* **170**, 793–798.

Nielsen, R. and Huelsenbeck, J. P. 2002. Detecting positively selected amino acid sites using posterior predictive P-values. In *Pacific symposium on biocomputing* (eds. R. B. Altman, A. K. Dunker, L. Hunter, K. Lauderdale, and T. E. Klein). River Edge, NJ: World Scientific, pp. 576–588.

Nizeyi, J. *et al.* 1999. Cryptosporidium sp. and Giardia sp. infections in mountain gorillas (*Gorilla gorilla beringei*) of the Bwindi Impenetrable National Park, Uganda. *J. Parasitol.* **85**, 1084–1088.

Noble, J. V. 1974. Geographic and temporal development of plague. *Nature* **250**, 726.

Normile, D. 2004. Mounting lab accidents raise SARS fears. *Science* **304**, 659–661.

Normile, D. and Enserink M. 2003. Tracking the roots of a killer. *Science* **301**, 297–299.

O'Neill, O. 2002*a*. *Autonomy and trust in bioethics.* Cambridge University Press.

O'Neill, O. 2002*b*. Some limits of informed consent. J. Med. Ethics **28**, 0–3.

Ontario Expert Panel on SARS and Infectious Disease Control: 2004. *For the Public's Health: A Plan of Action.* Government of Ontario, Canada.

Osterhaus, A. 2001. Catastrophes after crossing species barriers. *Phil. T. Roy. Soc. B* **356**, 791–793.

Parmenter, R. *et al.* 1993. The hantavirus epidemic in the southwest: rodent population dynamics and the implications for transmission of hantavirus-associated adult respiratory distress syndrome (HARDS) in the Four Corners region. *Sevilleta LTER Publ.* (University of New Mexico) **41**, 1–44.

Paterson, R. 2004. SARS returns to China. *Lancet Infect. Dis.* **4**, 64.

Patz, J. *et al.* 2002. Climate change: regional warming and malaria resurgence. *Nature* **420**, 627–628.

Patz, J. and Confalonieri, U. 2004. Human health: infectious and parasitic diseases. *Millenium ecosystem assessment. Conditions and trends.* Washington, DC: Island Press.

Patz, J. and Wolfe, N. 2002. Global ecological change and human health. In *Conservation medicine: ecological health in practice* (eds., A. Aguirre, R. Ostfeld, G. Tabor, C. House, and M. Pearl). Oxford: Oxford University Press, pp. 167–181.

Peiris, J. S. M. *et al.* 2003*a*. Coronavirus as a possible cause of severe acute respiratory syndrome. *Lancet* **361**, 1319–1325.

Peiris, J. S. M. *et al.* 2003*b*. Prospective study of the clinical progression and viral load of SARS-associated coronavirus pneumonia in a community outbreak. *Lancet* **361**, 1767–1772.

Peiris, J. S. M. *et al.* 2003*c*. Clinical progression and viral load in a community outbreak of coronavirus-associated SARS pneumonia: a prospective study. *Lancet* **361**, 1767–1772.

Peiris, J. S. M. *et al.* 2003*d*. The severe acute respiratory syndrome. *N. Engl. J. Med.* **349**, 2431–2441.

Peiris, J. S. M. *et al.* 2003*e*. Children with respiratory diseases associated with metapneumovirus in Hong Kong. *Emerg. Infect. Dis.* **6**, 628–633.

Peiris, J. S. M. *et al.* 2004. Re-emergence of fatal human influenza A subtype H5N1 disease. *Lancet* **363**, 617–619.

Peiris, J. S. M. *et al.* 1999. Human infection with influenza H9N2. *Lancet* **354**, 916–917.

Plotkin, J. B. *et al.* 2002. Hemagglutinin sequence clusters and the antigenic evolution of influenza A virus. *Proc. Natl. Acad. Sci. USA* **99**, 6263–6268.

Poon, L. L. *et al.* 2003*a*. Early diagnosis of SARS Coronavirus infection by real time RT-PCR. *J. Clin. Virol.* **28**, 233–238.

Poon, L. L. *et al.* 2003*b*. Rapid diagnosis of a coronavirus associated with severe acute respiratory syndrome (SARS). *Clin. Chem.* **49**, 953–955.

Posada, D. *et al.* 2002. Recombination in evolutionary genomics. *Ann. Rev. Gen.* **36**, 75–97.

Poutanen, S. M. *et al.* 2003. Identification of severe acute respiratory syndrome in Canada. *N. Eng. J. Med.* **348**, 1995–2005.

Reed, K. D. *et al.* 2004. The detection of monkeypox in humans in the Western Hemisphere. *N. Eng. J. Med.* **350**, 342–350.

Reid, A. H. *et al.* 1999. Origin and evolution of the 1918 'Spanish' influenza virus hemagglutinin gene. *Proc. Natl. Acad. Sci. USA* **96**, 1651–1656.

Reid, A. H. *et al.* 2003. Relationship of pre-1918 avian influenza HA and NP sequences to subsequent avian influenza strains. *Avian Dis.* **47**, 921–925.

Reiter, P. and Sprenger, D. 1987. The used tire trade: a mechanism for the worldwide dispersal of container-breeding mosquitoes. *J. Am. Mosquito Control Assoc.* **3**, 494–501.

Rest, J. S. and Mindell, D. P. 2003. SARS associated coronavirus has a recombinant polymerase and coronaviruses have a history of host-shifting. *Infect. Genet. Evol.* **3**, 219–225.

Riley, S. *et al.* 2003. Transmission dynamics of the etiological agent of SARS in Hong Kong: impact of public health interventions. *Science* **300**, 1961–1966.

Rimmelzwaan, G. F. *et al.* 2003. A primate model to study the pathogenesis of influenza A (H5N1) virus infection. *Avian Dis.* **47**, 931–933.

Rivers, T. M. 1937. Viruses and Koch's postulates. *J. Bacteriol.* **33**, 1–12.

Robertson, J. S. 1993. Clinical influenza virus and the embryonated hen's egg. *Rev. Med. Virol.* **3**, 97–106.

Robertson, E. *et al.* 2004. The psychosocial effects of being quarantined following exposure to SARS: A qualitative study of Toronto healthcare workers. *Can. J. Psychiatr.* **49**, 391–393.

Roberton, S. *et al.* 2003. Hunting and trading wildlife: an investigation into the wildlife trade in and around the Pu Mat National Park, Nghe An Province, Vietnam. SFNC Project Management Unit, Nghe An, Vietnam.

Roberton, S. *et al.* 2004. The illegal wildlife trade in Quang Nam Province: covert investigations by specially trained forest rangers. An unpublished report of the WWF MOSAIC Project and Quang Nam Forest Protection Department. Tam Ky Town, Vietnam.

Robinson, J. G. and Bennett, E. L. (Eds.) 2000. *Hunting for sustainability in tropical forests.* Columbia: Columbia University Press.

Rodo, X. *et al.* 2002. ENSO and cholera: a non-stationary link related to climate change? *Proc. Natl. Acad. Sci. USA* **20**, 12901–12906.

Rosling, L. and Rosling, M. 2003. Pneumonia causes panic in Guangdong province. *BMJ.* **326**, 416.

Rota, P. A. *et al.* 2003. Characterization of a novel coronavirus associated with severe acute respiratory syndrome. *Science* **300**, 1394–1399.

Rott, R. 1992. The pathogenic determinant of influenza virus. *Vet. Microbiol.* **33**, 303–310.

Royal Society. 2002. *Infectious diseases in livestock. Scientific questions relating to the transmission, prevention and control of epidemic outbreaks of infectious disease in livestock in Great Britain.* Policy document: 15/02. London: Royal Society.

Ruan, Y. J. *et al.* 2003. Comparative full-length genome sequence analysis of 14 SARS coronavirus isolates and common mutations associated with putative origins of infection. *Lancet* **361**, 1779–1785.

Salas, R. *et al.* 1991. Venezuelan haemorrhagic fever. *Lancet* **338**, 1033–1036.

Sanz, A. I. *et al.* 1999. Genetic variability of natural populations of cotton leaf curl geminivirus, a single-stranded DNA virus. *J. Mol. Evol.* **49**, 672–681.

SARS Expert Committee 2003. SARS in Hong Kong: from experience to action. October 2003.

Schliekelman, P. *et al.* 2001. Natural selection and resistance to HIV. *Nature* **411**, 545–546.

Schmidt, K. and Ostfeld, R. 2001. Biodiversity and the dilution effect in disease ecology. *Ecology* **82**, 609–619.

Scholtissek, C. 1990. Pigs as 'mixing vessels' for the creation of new pandemic influenza A viruses. *Med. Principles Pract.* **2**, 65–71.

Scholtissek, C. *et al.* 1978. On the origin of the human influenza virus subtypes H2N2 and H3N2. *J. Virol.* **87**, 13–20.

Scholtissek, C. *et al.* 1993a. Analysis of influenza-A virus nucleoproteins for the assessment of molecular genetic mechanisms leading to new phylogenetic virus lineages. *Arch. Virol.* **131**, 237–250.

Scholtissek, C. *et al.* 1993b. The role of swine in the origin of pandemic influenza. In *Options for the control of influenza, II* (eds. C. Hannoun, A. P. Kendal, H. D. Klenk and F. L. Ruben). Amsterdam: Elsevier, pp. 193–201.

Scholtissek, C. *et al.* 1998. Influenza in pigs and their role as the intermediate host. In *Textbook of influenza* (eds. K. G. Nicholson, R. G. Webster, and A. J. Hay). Oxford: Blackwell Science, pp. 137–145.

Schreiber, A. *et al.* 1989. *Weasels, civets, mongooses and their relatives; an action plan for the conservation of mustelids and viverrids.* Switzerland: IUCN, Gland.

Shalev, A. Y. *et al.* 1998. 'Prospective study of post-traumatic stress disorder and depression following trauma'. *Am. J. Psychiatr.* **155(630)**, 637.

Shen, Z. *et al.* 2004. Superspreading SARS events, Beijing, 2003. *Emerg. Infect. Dis.* **10**, 256–260.

Shortridge, K. F. 1992. Pandemic influenza: a zoonosis? *Semin. Resp. Infect.* **7**, 11–25.

Sierra, S. *et al.* 2000. Response of foot-and-mouth disease virus to increased mutagenesis. Influence of viral load and fitness in loss of infectivity. *J. Virol.* **74**, 8316–8323.

Simmons, G. *et al.* 2004. Characterization of severe acute respiratory syndrome-associated coronavirus (SARS-CoV) spike glycoprotein-mediated viral entry. *Proc. Natl. Acad. Sci. USA* **101**, 4240–4245.

Simpson, D. 1978. Viral haemorrhagic fevers of man. *Bull. WHO* **56**, 819–832.

Smith, D. L. *et al.* 2002. Predicting the spatial dynamics of rabies epidemics on heterogeneous landscapes. *Proc. Natl. Acad. Sci. USA*, **99**, 3668–3672.

Sokolov, V. E. *et al.* 1997. New species of Viverrid of the genus *Viverra* (Mammalia, Carnivora) from Vietnam. *Zoo. Zh.* **76**, 585–589.

Srikosamatara, S. *et al.* 1992. Wildlife trade in Lao PDR and between Lao PDR and Thailand. *Nat. Hist. Bull. Siam. Soc.* **40**, 1–47.

Stanhope, M. J. *et al.* 2004. Evidence from the evolutionary analysis of nucleotide sequences for a recombinant history of SARS-CoV. *Infect. Genet. Evol.* **4**, 15–19.

Stavrinides, J. and Guttman, D. S. 2004. Mosaic evolution of the Severe Acute Respiratory Syndrome coronavirus. *J. Virol.* **78**, 76–82.

Steinglass, P. and Gerrity, E. 1990. Natural disasters and post-traumatic stress disorder: Short-term versus long-term recovery in two disaster-affected communities. *J. Appl. Soc. Psychol.* **20(1746)**, 1765.

Stephenson, C. B. *et al.* 1999. Phylogenetic analysis of a highly conserved region of the polymerase gene from 11 coronaviruses and development of a consensus polymerase chain reaction assay. *Virus Res.* **60**, 181–189.

Stevens, J. *et al.* 2004. Structure of the uncleaved human H1 hemagglutinin from the extinct 1918 influenza virus. *Science* **303**, 1866–1870.

Strimmer, K. and von Haeseler, A. 1996. Quartet puzzling: a quartet maximum likelihood method for reconstructing tree topologies. *Mol. Biol. Evol.* **13**, 964–969.

Subbarao, K. *et al.* 1998. Characterization of an avian influenza A (H5N1) virus isolated from a child with a fatal respiratory illness. *Science* **279**, 393–396.

Sundin, E. C. and Horowitz, M. J. 2003. Horowitz's Impact of Event scale evaluation of 20 years of use. *Psychosom Med.* **65**, 870–876.

Surridge, A. *et al.* 1999. Striped rabbits in Southeast Asia. *Nature* **400**, 726.

Taubenberger, J. K. *et al.* 1997. Initial genetic characterization of the 1918 'Spanish' influenza virus. *Science* **275**, 1793–1796.

Tauxe, R. V. *et al.* 1995. Epidemic cholera in the New World: translating field epidemiology into new prevention strategies. *Emerg. Infect. Dis.* **1**, 141–146.

Taylor, J. L. *et al.* 1993. An outbreak of cholera in Maryland associated with imported commercial frozen fresh coconut milk. *J. Infect. Dis.* **167**, 1330–1335.

Thibault, M. and Blaney, S. 2003. The oil industry as an underlying factor in the bushmeat crisis in Central Africa. *Conserv. Biol.* **17**, 1807–1813.

Thiel, V. *et al.* 2003. Mechanisms and enzymes involved in SARS coronavirus genome expression. *J. Gen. Virol.* **84**, 2305–2315.

Timmins, R. J. *et al.* 1998. Status and conservation of the Giant Muntjac *Megamuntiacus vuquangensis* and notes on other muntjac species in Lao P.D.R. *Oryx* **32**, 59–67.

Truyen, U. *et al.* 1995. Evolution of the feline-subgroup parvoviruses and the control of canine host-range in vivo. *J. Virol.* **69**, 4702–4710.

Tsang, K. W. *et al.* 2003. A cluster of cases of severe acute respiratory syndrome in Hong Kong. *N. Engl. J. Med.* **348**: 1977–1985.

Turner, P. E. and Elena, S. F. 2000. Cost of host radiation in an RNA virus. *Genetics* **156**, 1465–1470.

Uchino, B. N. *et al.* 1996. The relationship between social support and physiological processes: A review with emphasis on underlying mechanisms and implications for health. *Psychol. Bull.* **119**, 488–531.

Vabret, A. F. *et al.* 2001. Direct diagnosis of human respiratory coronaviruses 229E and OC43 by the polymerase chain reaction. *J. Virol. Methods* **97**, 59–66.

van den Hoogen, B. G. *et al.* 2001. A newly discovered human pneumovirus isolated from young children with respiratory tract disease. *Nature Med.* **7**, 719–724.

Varia, M. *et al.* 2003. Investigation of a nosocomial outbreak of severe acute respiratory syndrome (SARS) in Toronto. *CMAJ* **169(4)**, 285–292.

Wallinga, J. and Teunis, P. 2004. Different epidemic curves for severe acute respiratory syndrome reveal similar impacts of control measured. *Am. J. Epidem.* **160**, 509–516.

Wallis, J. and Lee, K. 1999. Primate conservation: the prevention of disease transmission. *Int. J. Primatol.* **20**, 803–826.

Wang, P. *et al.* 2004. Expression cloning of functional receptor used by SARS coronavirus. *Biochem. Biophys. Res. Comm.* **315**, 439–444.

Watts, J. 2004. China culls wild animals to prevent new SARS threat. *Lancet* **363**, 134.

Webby, R. J. and Webster, R. G. 2004. Are we ready for pandemic influenza? *Science* **302**, 1519–1522.

Webster, R. G. *et al.* 1992. Evolution and ecology of influenza A viruses. *Microbiol. Rev.* **56**, 152–179.

Webster, R. G. 1998. Evolution and ecology of influenza viruses: interspecies transmission. In *Textbook of influenza* (eds. K. G. Nicholson, R. G. Webster, and A. J. Hay). Oxford: Blackwell Science, pp. 109–119.

Webster, R. G. 2004. Wet markets—a continuing source of severe acute respiratory syndrome and influenza? *Lancet* **363**, 234–236.

Weiss, R. A. 2001. The Leeuwenhoek lecture 2001. Animal origins of human infectious disease. *Philos. T. Roy. Soc. B* **356**, 957–977.

Whelan, S. and Goldman, N. 2001. A general empirical model of protein evolution derived from multiple protein families using a maximum-likelihood approach. *Mol. Biol. Evol.* **18**, 691–699.

WHO 1997. Division of Emerging and Other Communicable Diseases Surveillance and Control Annual Report 1997. Geneva: World Health Organization, 1998 (unpublished document WHO/EMC/98.2).

WHO 2000. Global outbreak alert and response: report of a WHO meeting. Geneva: World Health Organization (unpublished document WHO/CDS/CSR/200.3).

WHO 2002*a*. Global crisis—global solutions. Managing public health emergencies of international concern through the revised International Health Regulations. Geneva: World Health Organization (unpublished document WHO/CDS/CSR/AR/2002.4).

WHO 2002*b*. World Health Organization. Progress Report 2002: Global defence against the infectious disease threat. URL: www.who.int/infectious-disease-news/cds2002/

WHO 2003*a*. Global defence against the infectious disease threat. Geneva: WHO, pp. 74–79.

WHO 2003*b*. Severe acute respiratory syndrome, update 92—chronology of travel recommendations, areas with local transmission, at: www.who.int/csr/don/2003_07_01/en/

WHO 2003*c*. Acute Respiratory syndrome, China. *Wkly. Epidem. Rep.* **78**, 41–74.

WHO 2003*d*. Multicentre Collaborative Network for Severe Acute Respiratory Syndrome (SARS) Diagnosis. 2003*d*. A multicentre collaboration to investigate the cause of severe acute respiratory syndrome. *Lancet* **361**, 1730–1733.

WHO 2003*e*. Severe acute respiratory syndrome (SARS). *Wkly Epidem. Rec.* **78**, 81–83.

WHO 2003*f*. Consensus document on the epidemiology of severe acute respiratory syndrome (SARS). The Organization WHO/CDS/CSR/GAR/sars/en/2003. 11.2003. 11–28–0030.

WHO 2003*g*. Severe acute respiratory syndrome, update 96—Taiwan, China: SARS transmission interrupted in last outbreak area, at: www.who.int/csr/don/2003_07_01/en/

WHO 2003*h*. Revision of the International Health Regulations. Geneva, World Health Organization, (World Health Assembly resolution WHA56.28. Available from: URL: www.who.int/gb/EB_WHA/PDF/WHA56/ea56r28.pdf

WHO 2003*i*. Visit of WHO expert team to review the outbreak of atypical pneumonia in Guangdong Province, final report. Geneva: World Health Organization (unpublished document).

WHO 2003*j*. WHO issues a global alert about cases of atypical pneumonia, at: www.who.int/csr/sars/archive/2003_03_12/en/

WHO 2003*k*. SARS: lessons from a new disease. In: The world health report 2003: shaping the future. Geneva: World Health Organization.

WHO 2003*l*. World Health Organization issues emergency travel advisory, at: www.who.int/csr/sars/archive/2003_03_15/en/

WHO 2003*m*. First data on stability and resistance of SARS coronavirus compiled by members of the WHO multi-center laboratory network on SARS etiology and diagnosis. www.who.int/csr/sars/survival_2003_05_04/en/index.html

WHO 2003*n*. Severe Acute Respiratory Syndrome (SARS) in Singapore. 10 September 2003, at www.who.int/csr/don/2003_09_10/en

WHO 2003*o*. Severe Acute Respiratory Syndrome (SARS) in Taiwan, China. 17 December 2003, at www.who.int/csr/don/2003_12_17/en

WHO 2003*p*. New case of laboratory-confirmed SARS in Guangdong, China—update 5. 31 January 2004, at www.who.int/csr/don/2004_01_31/en

WHO 2004*a*. Avian influenza A (H5N1). *Wkly. Epidem. Rec.* **79**, 65–70.

WHO 2004*b*. New case of laboratory-confirmed SARS in Guangdong, China–update 5, Vol. 2004. Geneva: World Health Organization.

WHO International Health Regulations (1969). Available from URL:www.who.int

Woelk, C. H. and Holmes, E. C. 2002. Reduced positive selection in vector-borne RNA viruses. *Mol. Biol. Evol.* **19**, 2333–2336.

Wolpe, P. R. 1998. The triumph of autonomy in American bioethics: a sociological view. In *Bioethics and society: constructing the ethical*, (eds. R. DeVries and J. Subedi). New Jersey NJ: Prentice Hall, pp 38–59.

Woolhouse, M. E. J. *et al.* 2001. Population biology of multihost pathogens. *Science* **292**, 1109–1112.

Woolhouse, M. E. J. 2002. Population biology of emerging and re-emerging pathogens. *Trends Microbiol.* **10**, S3–S7.

Worobey, M. *et al.* 2002. Questioning the evidence for genetic recombination in the 1918 "Spanish flu" virus. *Science* **296**, 211.

Worobey, M. and Holmes, E. C. 1999. Evolutionary aspects of recombination in RNA viruses. *J. Gen. Virol.* **80**, 2535–2544.

Wu, H. S. *et al.* 2004. Serologic and molecular biologic methods for SARS-associated coronavirus infection: Taiwan. *Emerg. Infect. Dis.* **10**, 304–310.

Xiao, Z. L. *et al.* 2003. A retrospective study of 78 patients with severe acute respiratory syndrome. *Chin. Med. J.* **116**, 805–810.

Xu, R.-H. *et al.* 2004. Epidemiologic clues to SARS origin in China. *Emerg. Infect. Dis.* www.cdc.gov/ncidod/EID/vol10no6/030852.htm

Yam, W. C. *et al.* 2003. Evaluation of reverse transcription-PCR assays for rapid diagnosis of severe acute respiratory syndrome associated with a novel coronavirus. *J. Clin. Micro.* **41**, 4521–4524.

Yang, Z. *et al.* 2000. Codon-substitution models for heterogeneous selection pressure at amino acid sites. *Genetics* **155**, 431–449.

Yang, Z. 2000. Maximum likelihood estimation on large phylogenies and analysis of adaptive evolution in human influenza virus A. *J. Mol. Evol.* **51**, 423–432.

Yang, Z. Y. *et al.* 2004. A DNA vaccine induces SARS coronavirus neutralization and protective immunity in mice. *Nature* **428**, 561–564.

Yeh, S. H. *et al.* 2004. Characterization of severe acute respiratory syndrome coronavirus genomes in Taiwan: molecular epidemiology and genome evolution. *Proc. Natl. Acad. Sci. USA* **101**, 2542–2547.

Yu, D. *et al.* 2003. *MMWR Morb. Mortal. Wkly. Rep.* 52: 986–987.

Zambon, M. 2004. The inexact science of influenza prediction. *Lancet* **363**, 582–583.

Zheng, B. J. *et al.* 2004. SARS related virus predating SARS outbreak, Hong Kong. *Emerg. Infec. Dis.* **10**, 176–178.

Zhong, N. S. *et al.* 2003. Epidemiology and cause of severe acute respiratory syndrome (SARS) in Guangdong, People's Republic of China, in February, 2003. *Lancet* **362**, 1355–1358.

Zhong, N. S. 2004. Management and prevention of SARS in China. *Philos. T. Roy. Soc. B* **359**, 1115–1116.

Zhong, N. S. and Zeng, G. Q. 2003. Our strategies for fighting severe acute respiratory syndrome (SARS). *Am. J. Resp. Dis. Crit. Care Med.* **168**, 7–9.

Zhou, L. X. *et al.* 2003. The index case of SARS in Foshan, Guangdong Province. *Chin. J. Tuber. and Respir. Dis.* **26**, 598–601.

Index

Page numbers in *italics* refer to Tables and Figures. No references are given under 'SARS' or 'SARS-CoV', as these cover most of the book. Readers are advised to search under a more specific heading.